Atlas of Orthopaedic Surgical Approaches to the Lower Limbs

Rosa Ballis • Bujar H. Shabani • Dafina Bytyqi

Atlas of Orthopaedic Surgical Approaches to the Lower Limbs

Springer

Rosa Ballis
Department of Orthopedics
Ospedale S.Martino Belluno
Belluno, Italy

Dafina Bytyqi
Faculty of Medicine, University of Prishtina
Prishtina, Kosovo

Bujar H. Shabani
Faculty of Medicine, University of Prishtina
Prishtina, Kosovo

ISBN 978 3 031 07725 8 ISBN 978-3-031-07723-4 (eBook)
https://doi.org/10.1007/978-3-031-07723-4

This Springer imprint is published by the registered company Springer Nature Switzerland AG
The registered company address is: Gewerbestrasse 11, 6330 Cham, Switzerland

For all those who believed in me
Rosa Ballis

To our family
Bujar Shabani, Dafina Bytyqi

Preface

It is believed that the surgery, besides being based on science and evidence-based data and precision, it is an ART also. This book proves that there is an artistic side on a surgeon. The drawings you will find here were made by the author Dr. Rosa Ballis, an orthopedic surgeon and artist. The style in anatomy drawing came from the greatest anatomist from the past like Andrea Vesalio and watercolors emphasized the importance of every single anatomical structure and transmit the flow of the surgical procedure. The pictures came from the direct experience on the surgical field and some dissection taken in ICLO Verona. This book has been written primarily for orthopaedic residents as a manual, to introduce the most common approaches to the lower limb, but could be worth reading for medical students and other healthcare professionals. The text added to the drawings is short and concise, straight to the point, in order to make it easy and understandable for the reader. Each section, Hip, Knee and Ankle starts with anatomy chapter which explains most important structures. Each approach has an introduction which points out the indications and then step by step progress to the structure aimed. We wish you enjoy this book as much as we did writing it!

Belluno, Italy — Rosa Ballis
Prishtina, Kosovo — Bujar H. Shabani
Prishtina, Kosovo — Dafina Bytyqi

Acknowledgements

I would like to thank my colleagues for the useful suggestions and the patience to permit the drawing of every single step of the surgical procedures.

Thanks to Grezda Kushtrim, orthopaedics resident, and his contribution in some sections in the book.

I would like to thank my colleague Syed Hassan for the language revision.

Contents

Part II Knee

Part III Tibia and Fibula

Part I

Hip and Femur

1 Anatomy of the Hip

1.1 Introduction

Hip is one of the largest joints in the body. It is a ball-socket joint that allows a lot of movement but also carries the weight of the body. Hip is one of the most operated joint, from simple arthrotomies, fracture fixations, joint replacements to complex tumor resections and reconstructions. Because the hip is a deep structure, surrounded by a thick envelope of muscles and important neurovascular structures pass around the area, multiple approaches have been utilized to exposure the joint. The knowledge of anatomy and important landmarks is essential to choose the most convenient and safe approach and to avoid unnecessary damage to soft tissue structures. In this chapter, you will find he most important structures involved in surgical approaches to the hip and femur. Muscles, arteries and nerves are easily identifiable through simple captions.

R. Ballis et al., *Atlas of Orthopaedic Surgical Approaches to the Lower Limbs*, https://doi.org/10.1007/978-3-031-07723-4_1

1.2 Muscles

1.2.1 Anterior View

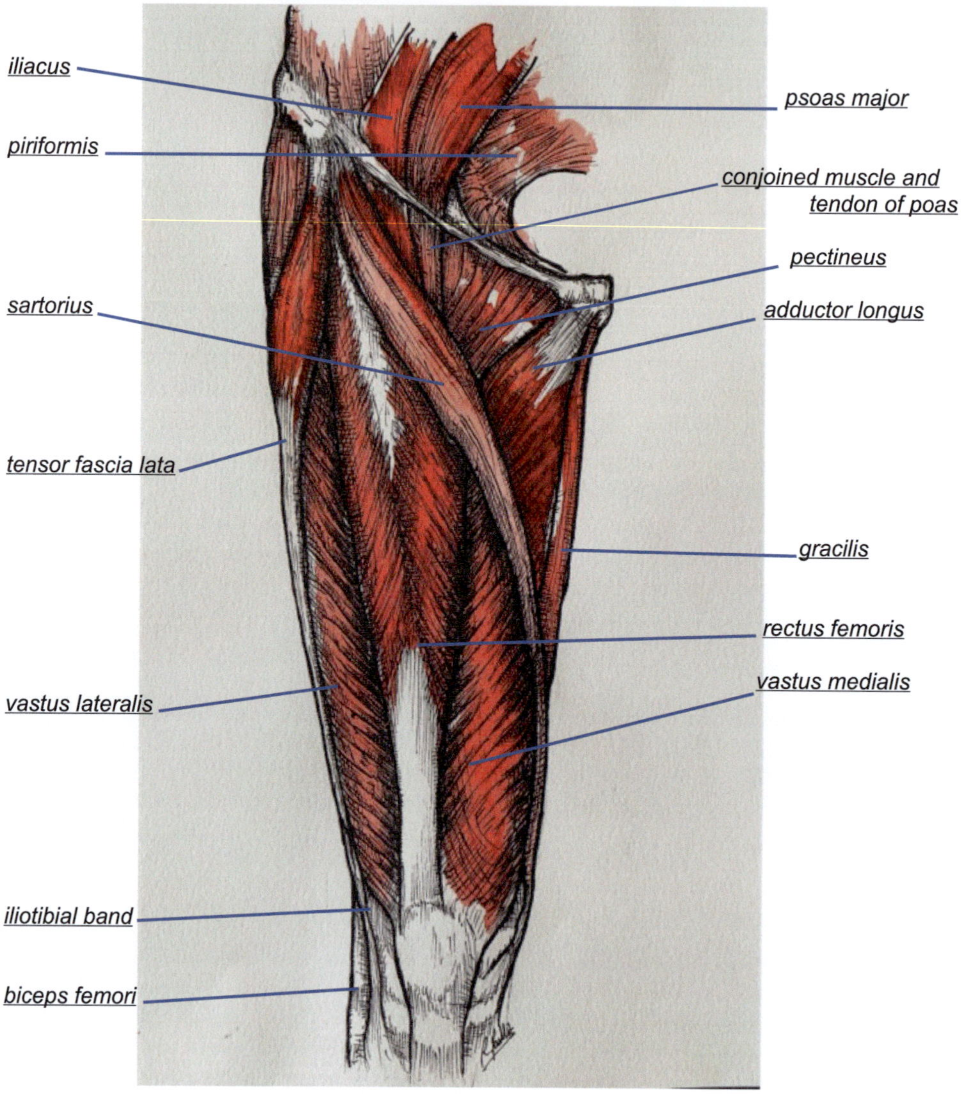

1.2.2 Lateral View

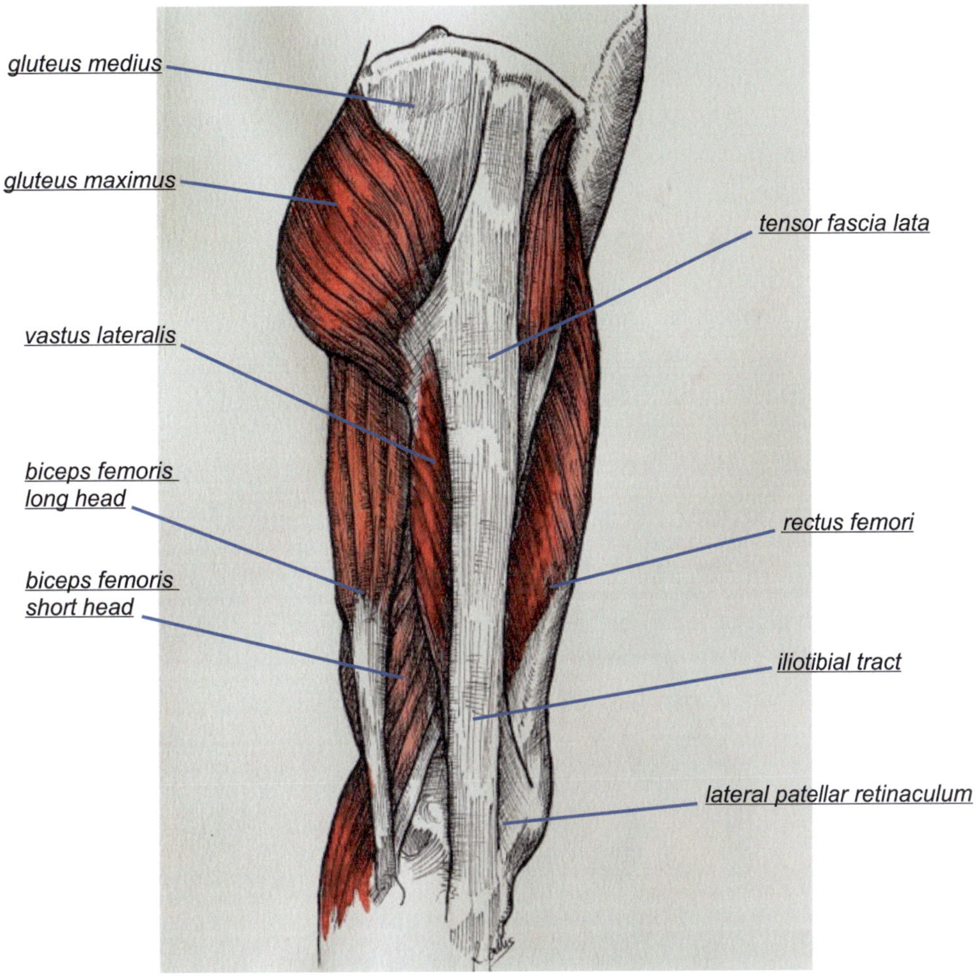

1.2.3 Posterior View

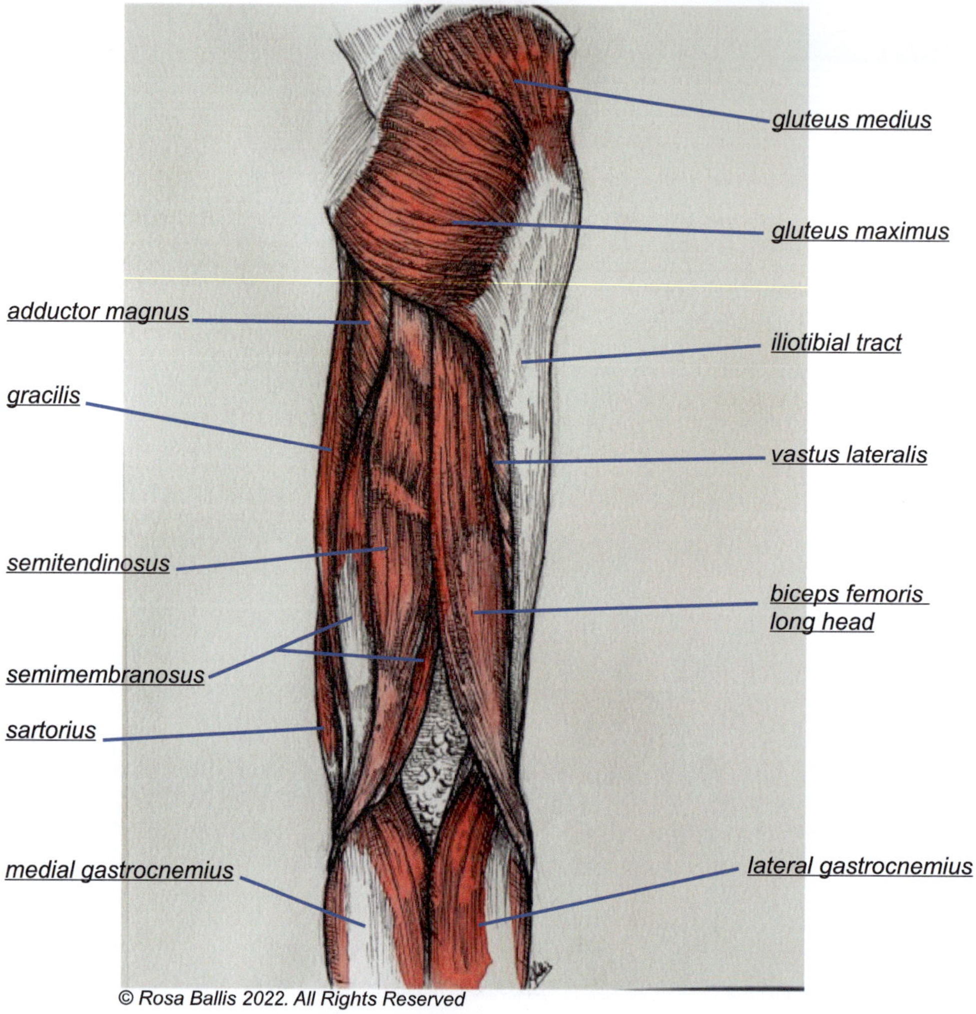

1.3 Nerves

1.3.1 Anterior View

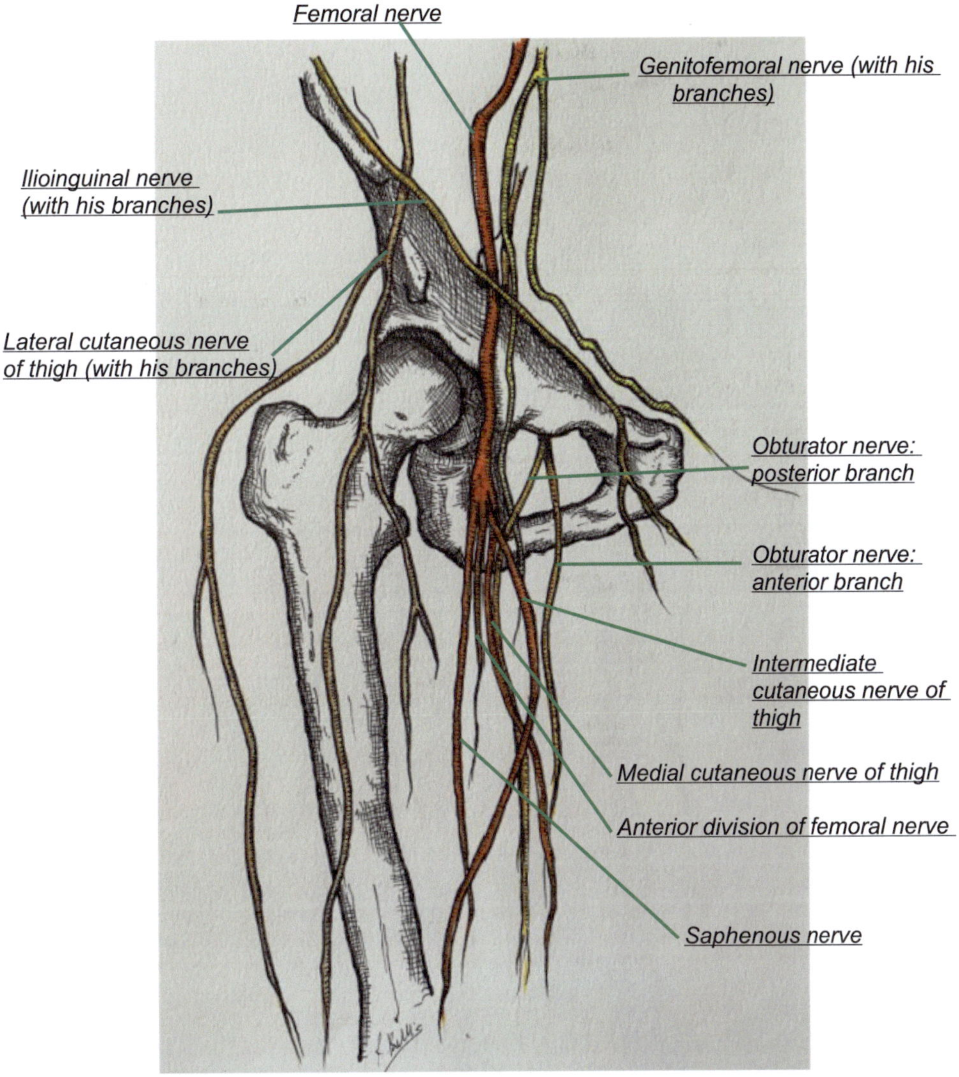

1.3.2 Posterior View

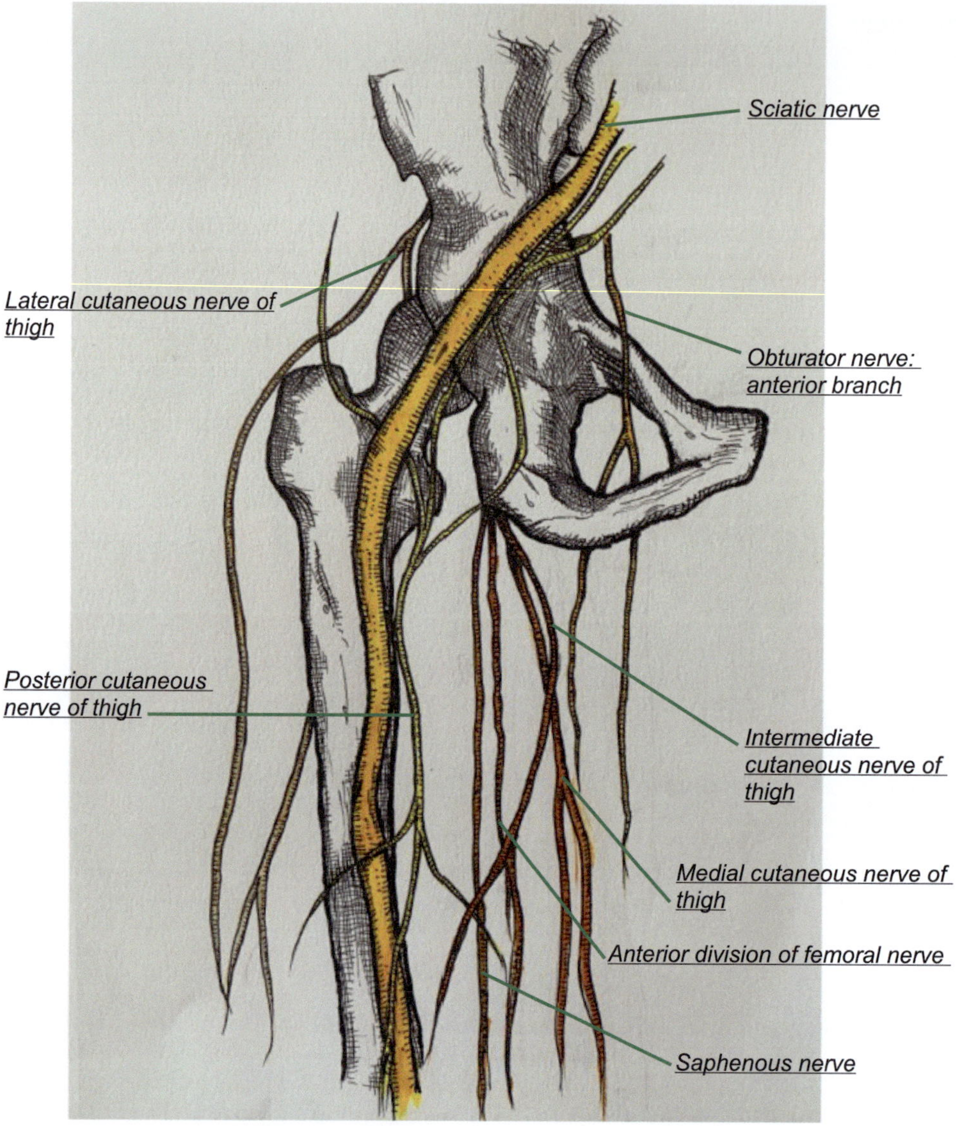

1.4 Arteries

1.4.1 Anterior View

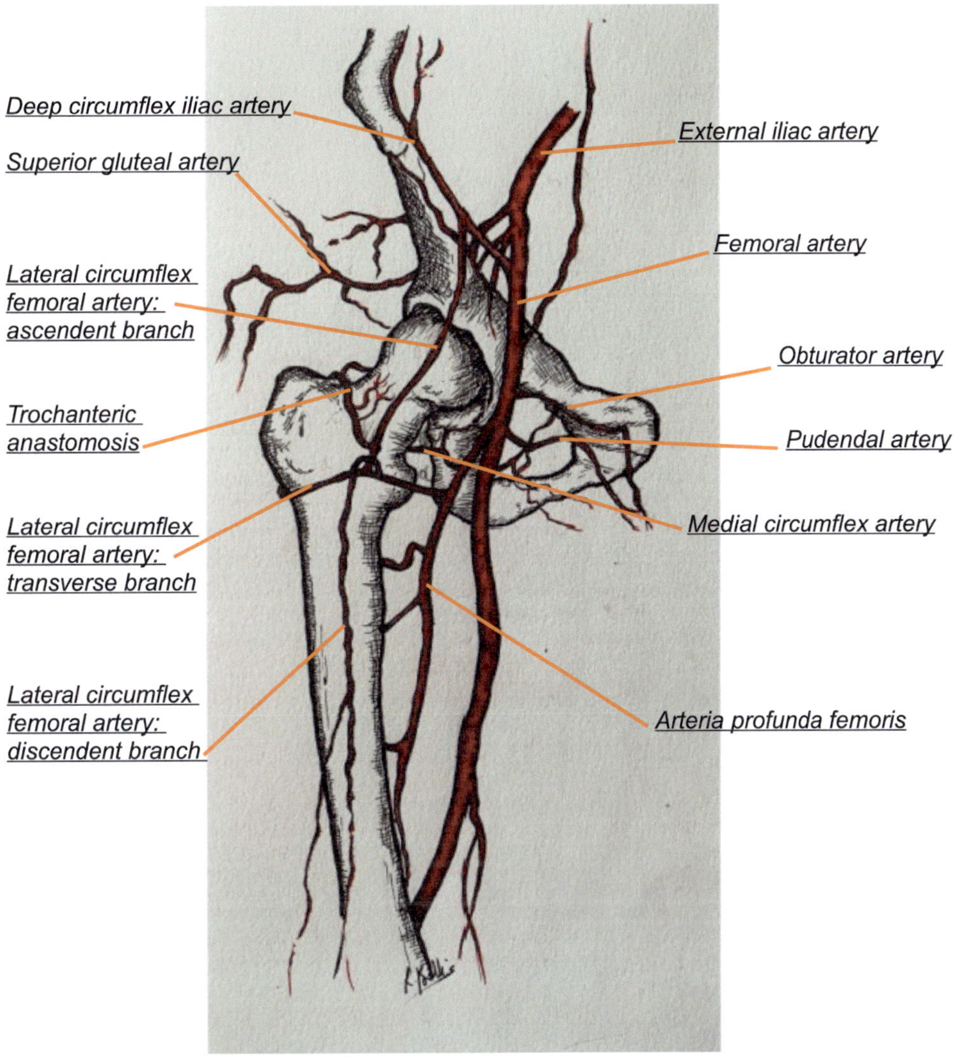

1.4.2 Posterior View

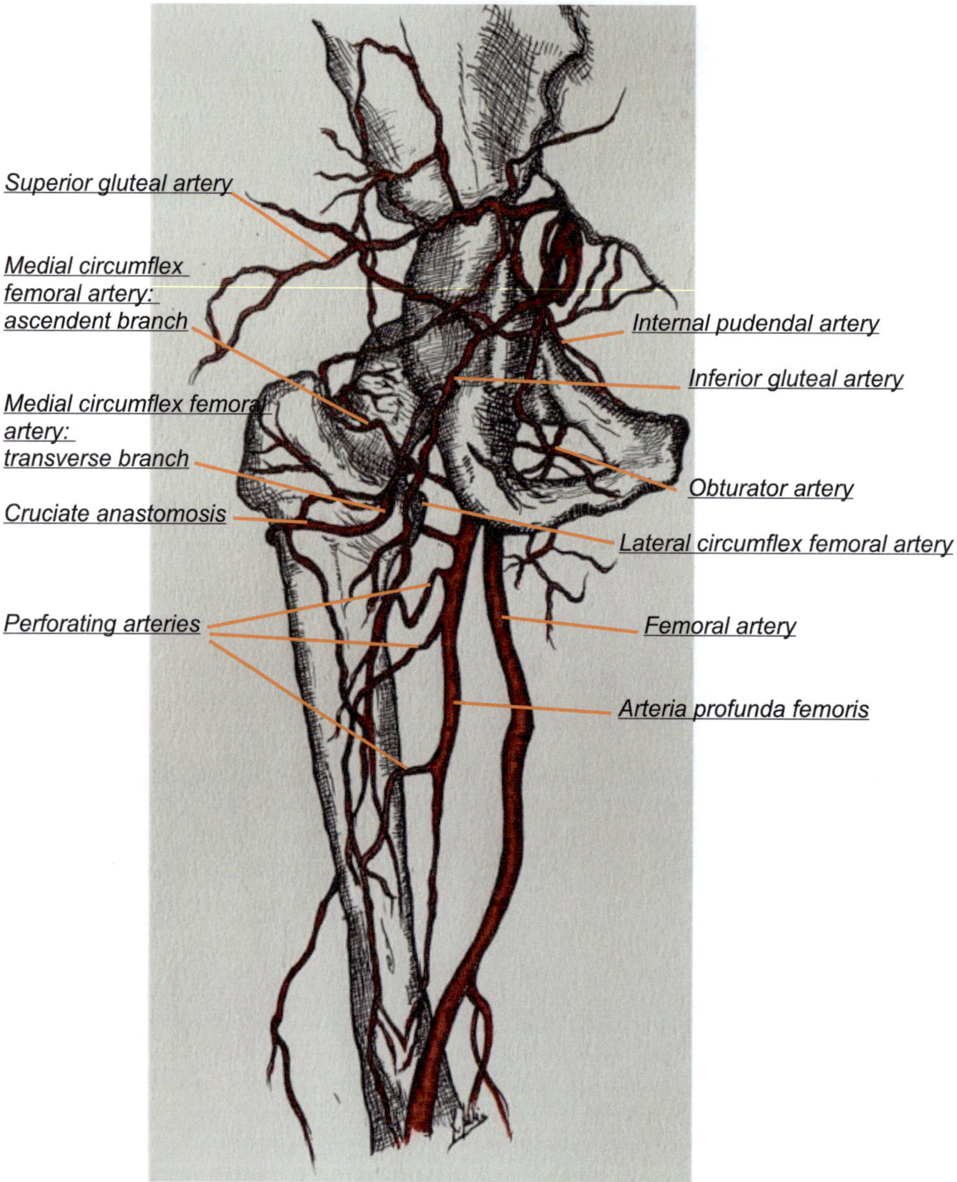

Anterolateral Approach to the Hip: Watson-Jones

2

2.1 Introduction

This approach has been used widely lately. At first, fascia lata and gluteus medius (GM) were cut during this approach but now, an intermuscular interval is used between tensor fascia lata and GM.

- Indications: Total hip replacement; hemiarthroplasty; ORIF (Open Reduction Internal Fixation), synovial biopsy, bone biopsy.
- Position of the patient: Usually the patient should be in supine position (reduces pelvic tilt). Could be performed also in lateral decubitus.
- Landmarks: (1) Anterior superior iliac spine (ASIS); (2) greater trochanter, (3) shaft of the femur.

2.2 Step-by-Step Procedure

Incision: Starts just posterior to ASIS, curves posteriorly and distally along 1\3 of anterior margin of trochanter before running down to the shaft of the femur (Fig. 2.1).

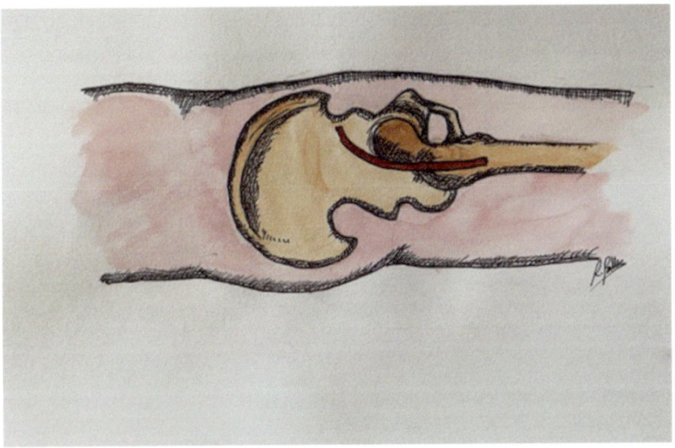

Fig. 2.1 Landmarks and incision. (© Rosa Ballis 2022. All Rights Reserved)

R. Ballis et al., *Atlas of Orthopaedic Surgical Approaches to the Lower Limbs*, https://doi.org/10.1007/978-3-031-07723-4_2

Incision of fascia lata should be made over trochanter, than from distal to proximal, remaining anterior to the gluteus medius muscle (Fig. 2.2).

The interval between tensor fascia lata and gluteus medius is developed by blunt dissection (Fig. 2.3). Care should be taken to not extend the gluteus medius split more than 5 cm proximal to the tip of greater trochanter to avoid damaging the superior gluteal nerve.

A retractor is placed anteriorly over the hip capsule, often in the superior part of the acetabulum (Fig. 2.4).

External rotation of the leg improves access to the hip capsule.

The capsule is incised after the hip was externally rotated to put the capsule on stretch (Fig. 2.5).

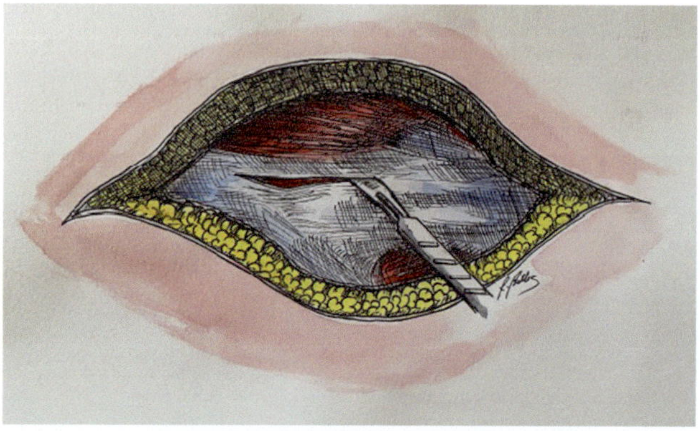

Fig. 2.2 Incision of fascia lata. (© Rosa Ballis 2022. All Rights Reserved)

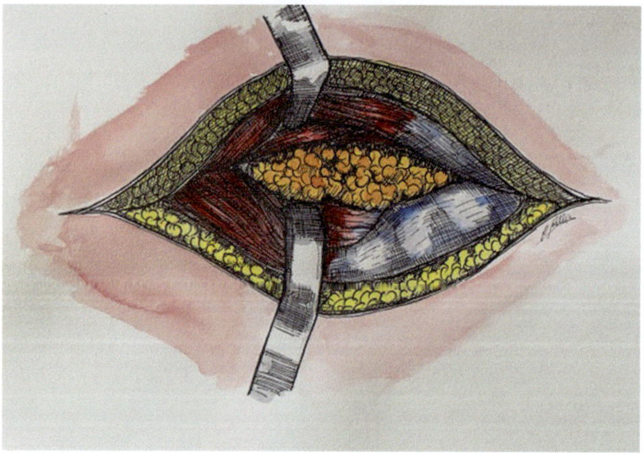

Fig. 2.3 Intermuscular dissection. (© Rosa Ballis 2022. All Rights Reserved)

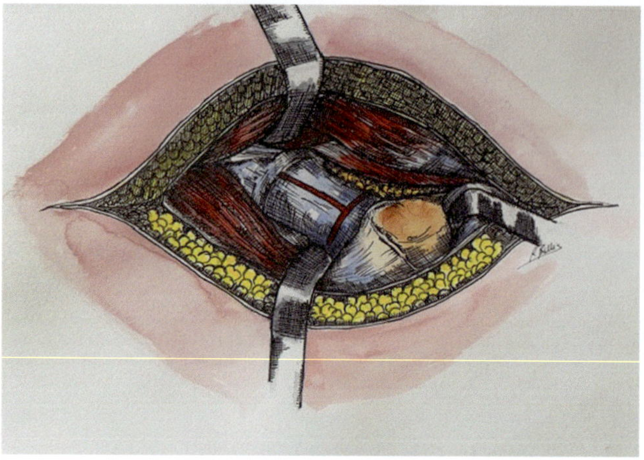

Fig. 2.4 Capsule exposure. (© Rosa Ballis 2022. All Rights Reserved)

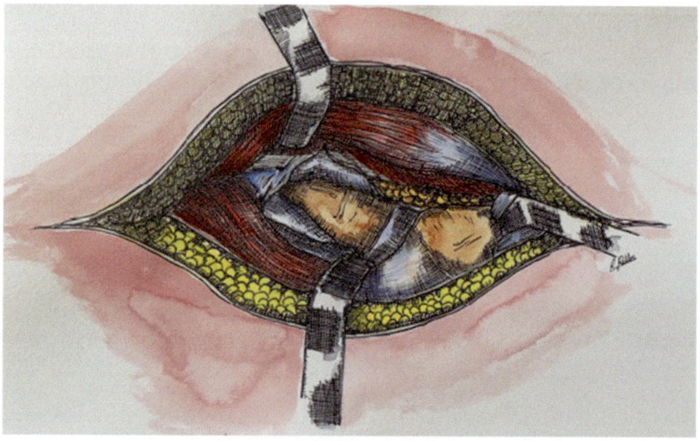

Fig. 2.5 Capsule incision. (© Rosa Ballis 2022. All Rights Reserved)

2.3 Structures at Risk

- Superior gluteal nerve remains a potential risk during gluteus medius split.
- Femoral nerve, artery and vein can be damaged during medial retraction.

3 Anterior Approach to the Hip: Smith-Petersen

3.1 Introduction

Anterior approach provides the direct access to the hip joint and for many surgeons it is more challenging. The muscles are bluntly separated and are spared from damage but there are neuro-vascular structures that need to be protected and addressed.

- Indications: Total hip replacement; hemiarthroplasty; reduction of femoral head and neck fractures; synovial biopsy, bone biopsy; pelvic osteotomies; intraarticular fusion; draining infections.
- Position of the patient: Supine position (reduces pelvic tilt).

3.2 Step-by-Step Procedure

Incision: Below ASIS running distally parallel to sartorius muscle (Fig. 3.1).

The interval between tensor fascia lata (TFL) and sartorius needs to be identified.

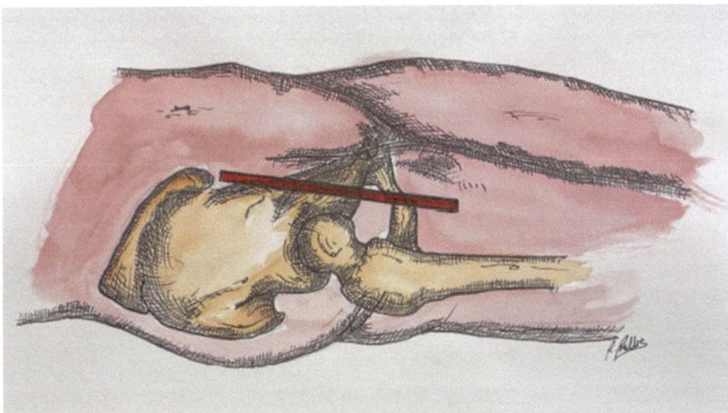

Fig. 3.1 Incision. (© Rosa Ballis 2022. All Rights Reserved)

R. Ballis et al., *Atlas of Orthopaedic Surgical Approaches to the Lower Limbs*, https://doi.org/10.1007/978-3-031-07723-4_3

Incision of the fascia should be made by caution because of lateral cutaneous nerve (it must be exposed and retracted medially) (Fig. 3.2).

Blunt finger dissection is utilized and the interval between TFL and sartorius is developed. Ascending branch of lateral femoral circumflex artery should be identified (Fig. 3.3).

Rectus femoris is identified and released from the anterior inferior iliac spine then retracted medially. Gluteus medius is retracted laterally and hip capsule exposed. Ascending branch of circumflex artery should be ligated (Fig. 3.4).

Capsule is then identified and a capsulotomy is done (Figs. 3.5 and 3.6).

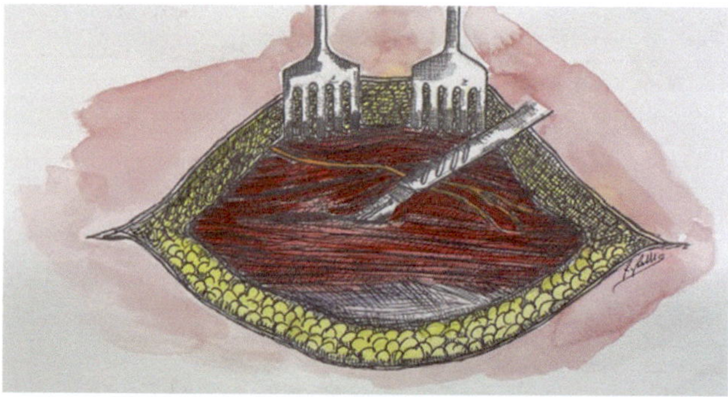

Fig. 3.2 Incision of tensor fascia and nerve identification. (© Rosa Ballis 2022. All Rights Reserved)

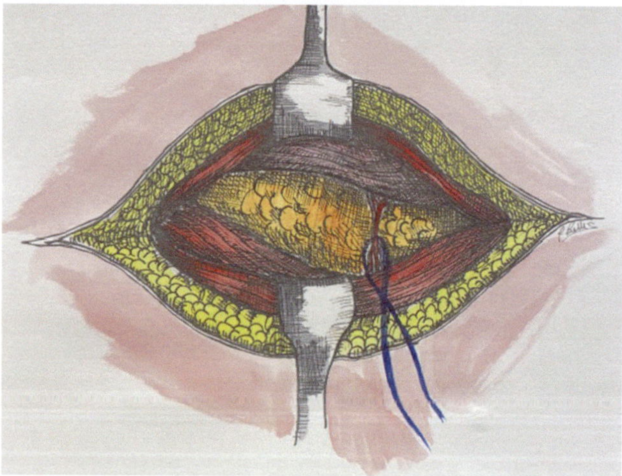

Fig. 3.3 Deep surgical dissection: interval between tensor fascia lata and sartorius. Identification of branch of circumflex artery. (© Rosa Ballis 2022. All Rights Reserved)

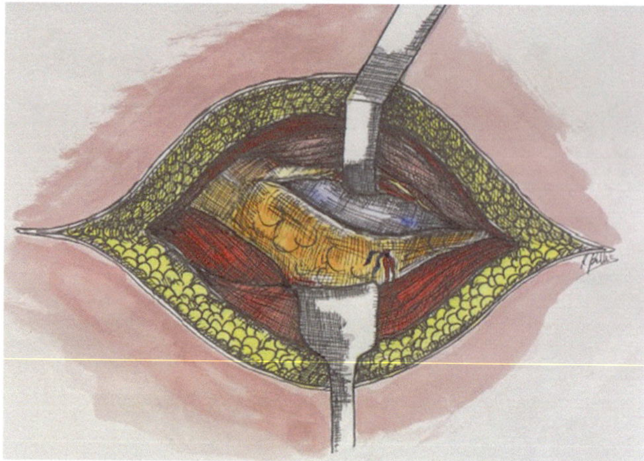

Fig. 3.4 Ligation of branch of circumflex artery and capsule identification. (© Rosa Ballis 2022. All Rights Reserved)

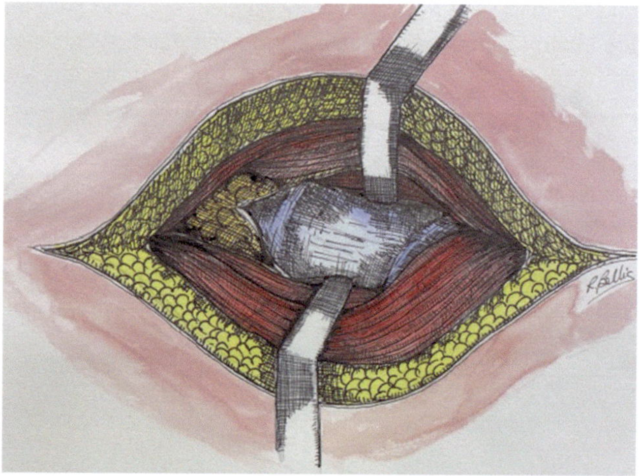

Fig. 3.5 Capsule exposure. (© Rosa Ballis 2022. All Rights Reserved)

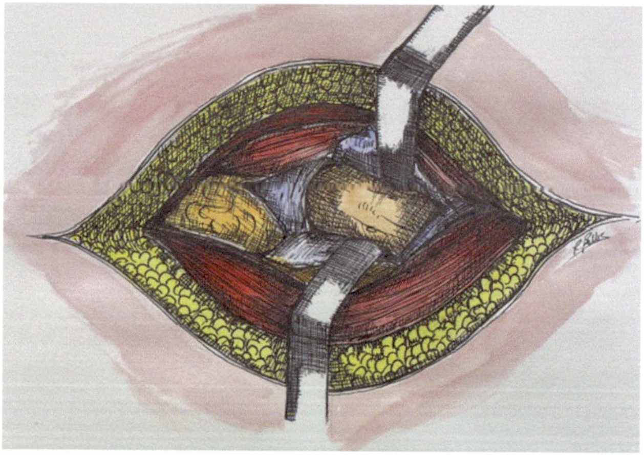

Fig. 3.6 Capsulotomy. (© Rosa Ballis 2022. All Rights Reserved)

3.3 Structures at Risk

- Lateral femoral cutaneous nerve
- Femoral nerve (dissection must be taken lateral to sartorius)
- Ascending branch of lateral femoral circumflex artery

4 Direct Lateral Approach to the Hip: Hardinge

4.1 Introduction

Lateral approach of the hip is commonly used. It involves the release of abductors, which may affect the gait afterwards.

- Indications: Hemiarthroplasty, primary total hip arthroplasty, proximal femur fracture.
- Position of the patient: Lateral, supine.

4.2 Step-by-Step Procedure

Incision: 3–5 cm proximal to tip of greater trochanter. The incision goes distally over the greater trochanter and extends down to the line of the femur (Fig. 4.1).

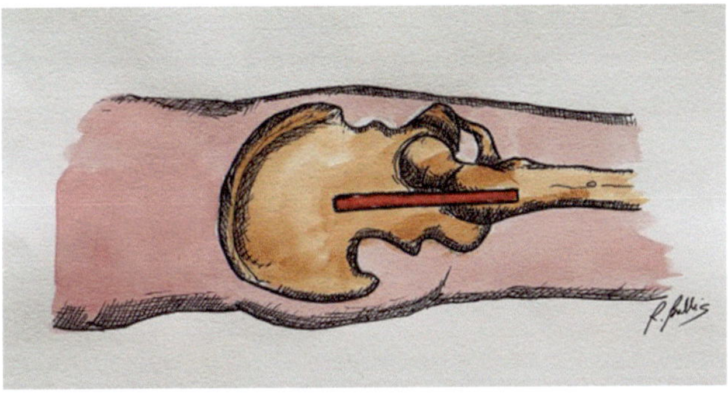

Fig. 4.1 Incision. (© Rosa Ballis 2022. All Rights Reserved)

R. Ballis et al., *Atlas of Orthopaedic Surgical Approaches to the Lower Limbs*, https://doi.org/10.1007/978-3-031-07723-4_4

First fascia lata must be splitted proximally until its muscular portion (Fig. 4.2).

Gluteus medius and vastus lateralis muscles are exposed (Fig. 4.3).

Gluteus medius is splitted longitudinally from the middle of greater trochanter and approach extended through fibers of vastus lateralis. It is important to preserve posterior insertion of gluteus medius (Fig. 4.4).

A T-shaped capsulotomy must be made to expose the joint (Fig. 4.5).

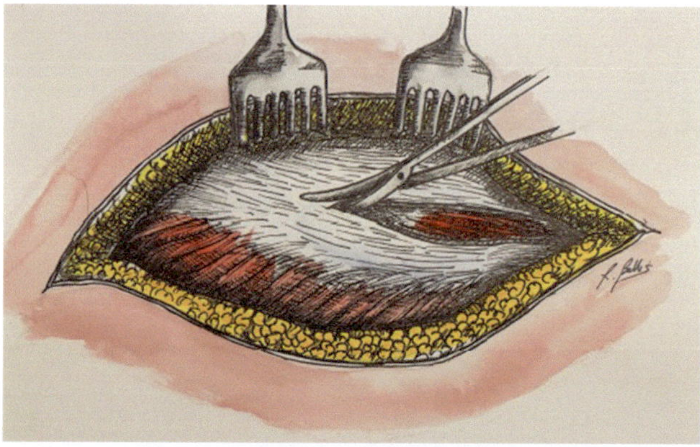

Fig. 4.2 Fascia lata splitting. (© Rosa Ballis 2022. All Rights Reserved)

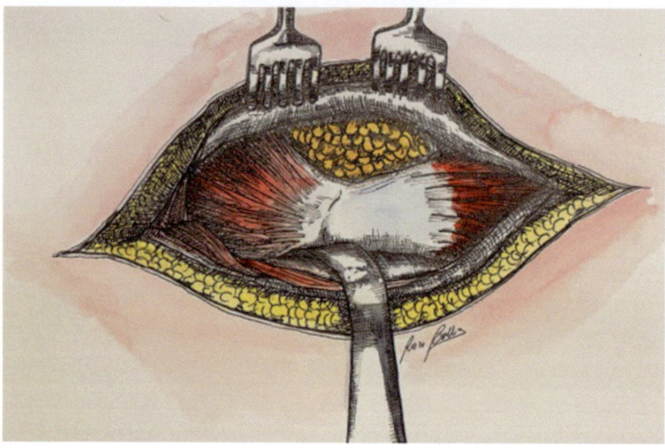

Fig. 4.3 Gluteus medius and vastus lateralis exposed. (© Rosa Ballis 2022. All Rights Reserved)

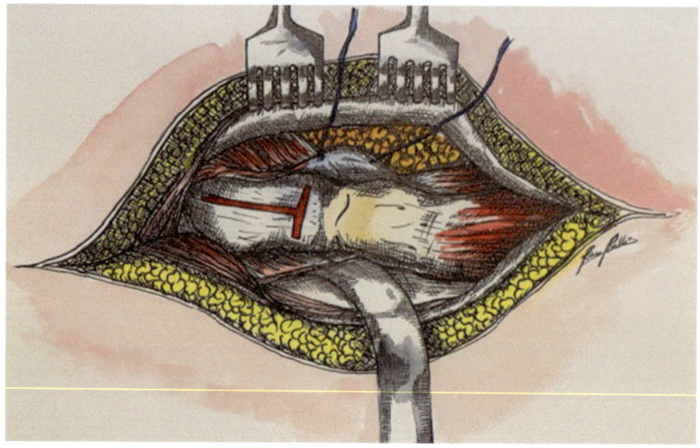

Fig. 4.4 Gluteus medius release and capsule exposure. (© Rosa Ballis 2022. All Rights Reserved)

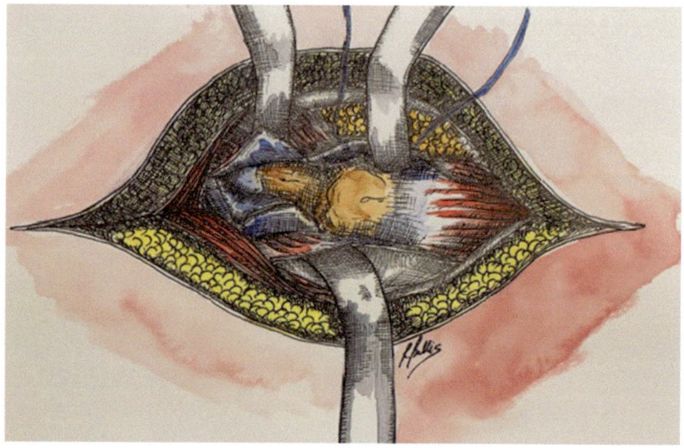

Fig. 4.5 Joint exposure. (© Rosa Ballis 2022. All Rights Reserved)

4.3 Structure at Risk

- Superior gluteal nerve (proximal incision has to be limited 3–5 cm from greater trochanter)
- Femoral nerve (retractors must be kept on bone to prevent iatrogenic injury)

5 Posterolateral Approach to the Hip: Moore

5.1 Introduction

Posterolateral approach provides great exposure of proximal femur and acetabulum. It is considered as simple and relatively easy to learn, and it is the most used approach for Total Hip Replacement. External rotators are dissected for exposure.

- Indications: Total hip replacement; revision THA; periprosthetic femur fracture; periprosthetic acetabular fracture; acetabular fracture.
- Position of the patient: Lateral decubitus; prone position (in the transverse acetabular fracture).

5.2 Step-by-Step Procedure

Incision: Incision is started 6 cm proximal and posterior to the lateral side of greater trochanter (Fig. 5.1). The incision is continued down to the shaft of femur in the midline.

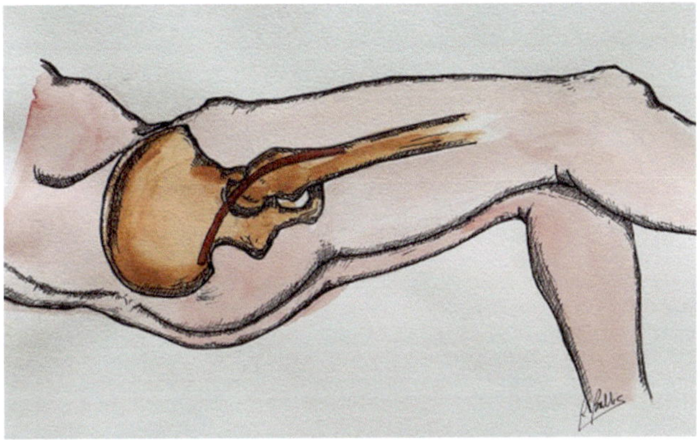

Fig. 5.1 Lateral decubitus of patient and incision. (© Rosa Ballis 2022. All Rights Reserved)

R. Ballis et al., *Atlas of Orthopaedic Surgical Approaches to the Lower Limbs*, https://doi.org/10.1007/978-3-031-07723-4_5

After fascia lata dissection, vastus lateralis muscle and gluteal muscle are exposed (Fig. 5.2).

The leg is placed on internal rotation before continuing dissection (Fig. 5.3).

Gluteus muscle flap is retracted posteriorly and external rotators are shown (Fig. 5.4).

Sutures must be done in the tendinous part of external rotators before dissecting them (Fig. 5.5).

T-shaped incision of the capsule (Fig. 5.6).

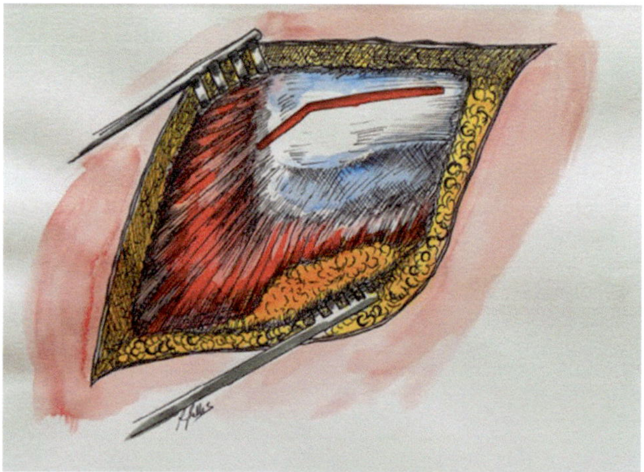

Fig. 5.2 Fascia lata incision. (© Rosa Ballis 2022. All Rights Reserved)

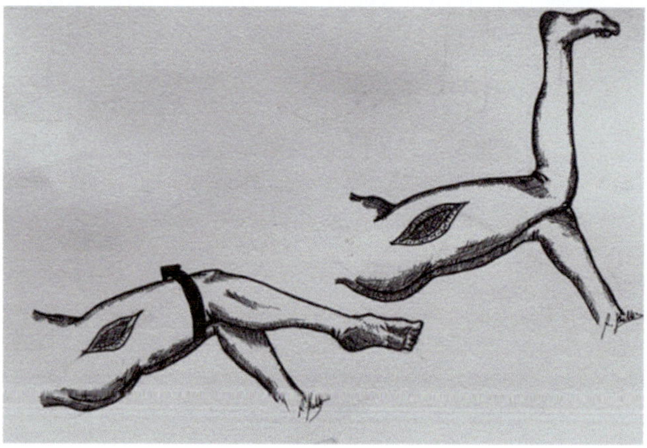

Fig. 5.3 Hip internal rotation to expose capsule and external rotator muscles. (© Rosa Ballis 2022. All Rights Reserved)

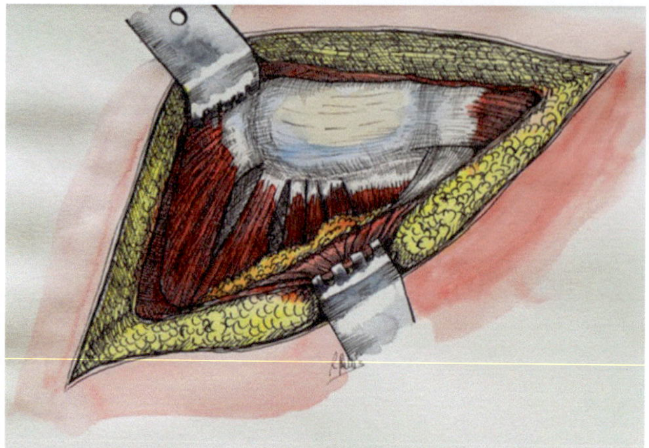

Fig. 5.4 External rotator muscles exposure. (© Rosa Ballis 2022. All Rights Reserved)

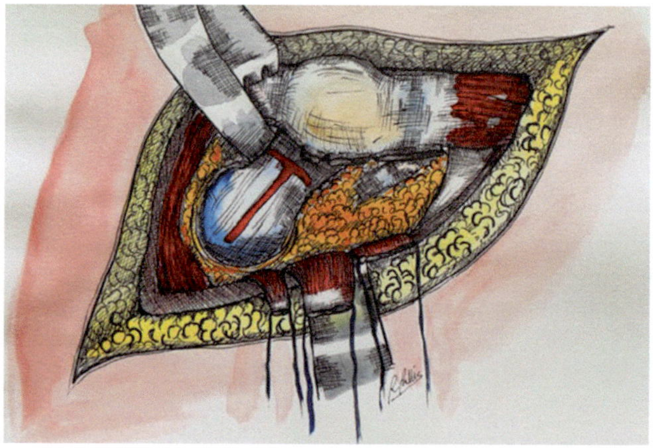

Fig. 5.5 Capsule incision. (© Rosa Ballis 2022. All Rights Reserved)

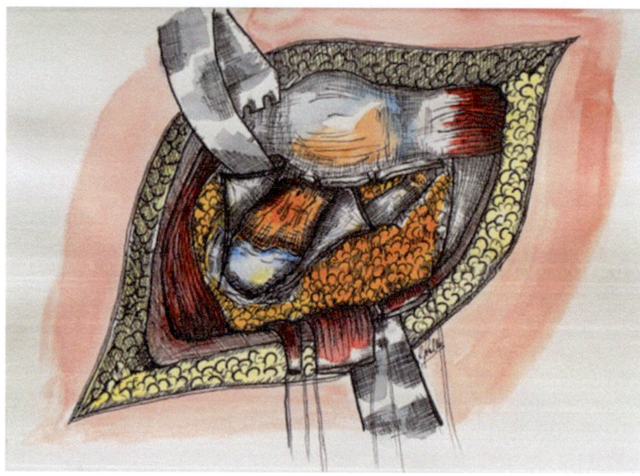

Fig. 5.6 Femoral neck exposure. (© Rosa Ballis 2022. All Rights Reserved)

5.3 Structures at Risk

- Sciatic nerve (hip needs to be extended and knee flexed to prevent injury)
- Superior gluteal nerve (if the split between gluteus maximus and medius is too far proximal)

6 Lateral Approach to the Femur

6.1 Introduction

Lateral approach of the femur is used mainly for fractures of the proximal femur. Because the main vessels are medial to femur, this approach is considered easy and safe.

- Indications: Fractures (peritrochanteric, intertrochanteric, subtrochanteric, femoral neck fracture, shaft fractures), periprosthetic fracture, subtrochanteric and intertrochanteric osteotomy, biopsy.
- Position of the patient: Supine (usually).

6.2 Step-by-Step Procedure

Incision: Greater trochanter, along the shaft of femur between the greater trochanter and the lateral femoral epicondyle (Fig. 6.1).

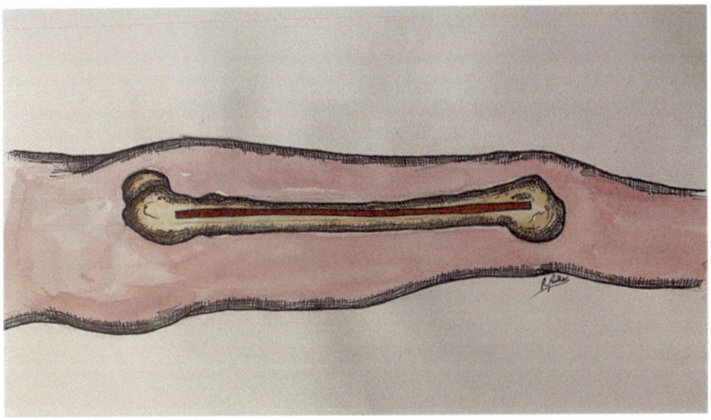

Fig. 6.1 Incision. © Rosa Ballis 2022. All Rights Reserved

R. Ballis et al., *Atlas of Orthopaedic Surgical Approaches to the Lower Limbs*, https://doi.org/10.1007/978-3-031-07723-4_6

The fascia lata is incised parallel to the skin incision (Fig. 6.2) and vastus lateralis muscle is exposed (Fig. 6.3).

Incision is brought through vastus lateralis, and the desired area of the femur is exposed. Vastus lateralis is incised about 1 cm anterior to the intermuscular septum (Fig. 6.4).

The muscle is retracted anteromedially. Care must be taken to identify the perforating vessels that needs to be ligated (Fig. 6.5).

Now shaft of femur is exposed (Fig. 6.6).

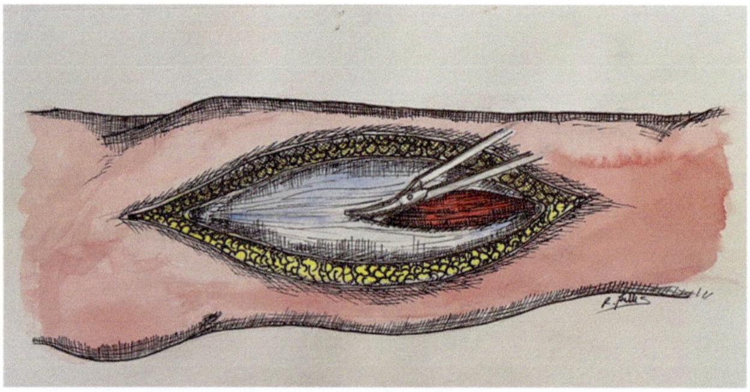

Fig. 6.2 Fascia lata release. © Rosa Ballis 2022. All Rights Reserved

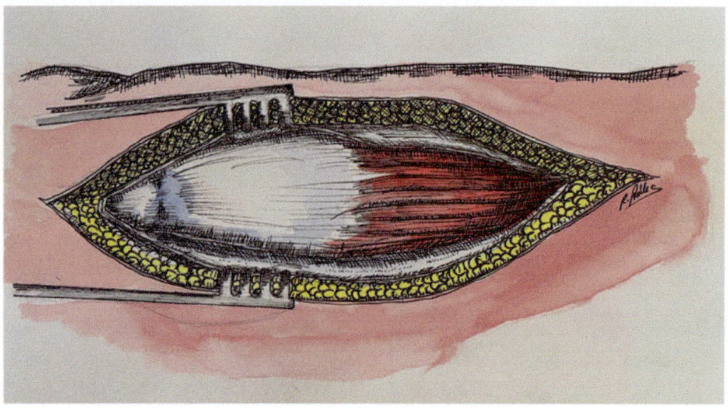

Fig. 6.3 Vastus lateralis muscle is exposed. © Rosa Ballis 2022. All Rights Reserved

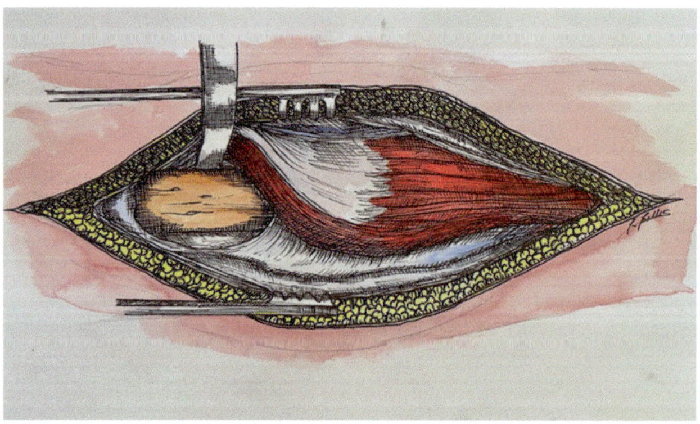

Fig. 6.4 Exposing femur. © Rosa Ballis 2022. All Rights Reserved

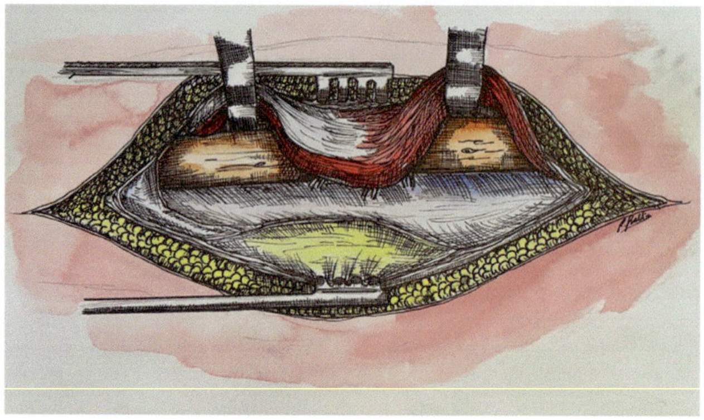

Fig. 6.5 Exposing different area of the femur. © Rosa Ballis 2022. All Rights Reserved

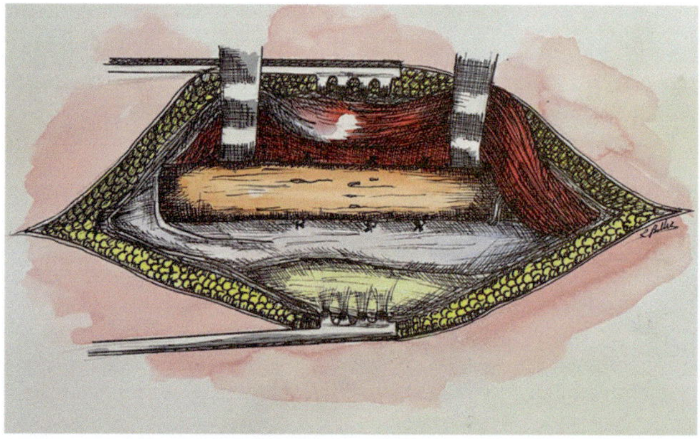

Fig. 6.6 Exposing the diaphysis and ligation of perforating arteries. © Rosa Ballis 2022. All Rights Reserved

6.3 Structure at Risk

- Perforating branches of the profunda femoris artery (should be ligated to prevent hematoma).

Lateral Distal Approach to the Femur

7

7.1 Introduction

Lateral distal femur approach is pretty straightforward and used for simple fractures of distal femur.

- Indications: Supracondylar fractures, iliotibial band release. It may be used in association with knee arthrotomies for articular fractures.
- Position of the patient: Supine with a support under the distal posterior thigh to defend the gastrocnemius forces.

7.2 Step-by-Step Procedure

Incision: Landmarks are midlateral line of the femoral shaft, Gerdy's tubercle and lateral femoral condyle (Fig. 7.1).

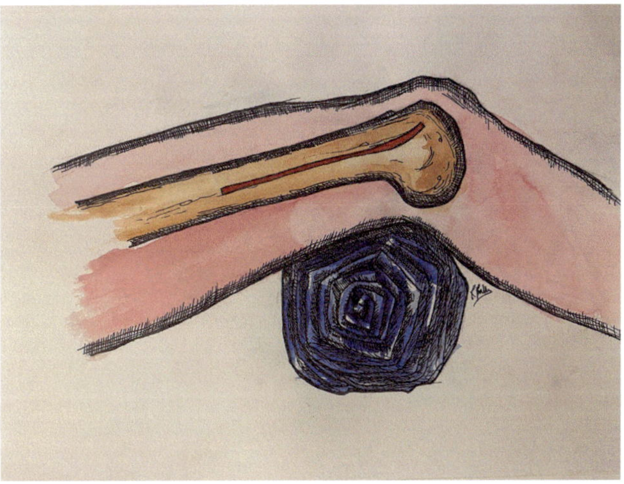

Fig. 7.1 Limb positioning and landmarks of incision. © Rosa Ballis 2022. All Rights Reserved

R. Ballis et al., *Atlas of Orthopaedic Surgical Approaches to the Lower Limbs*, https://doi.org/10.1007/978-3-031-07723-4_7

Incision of the fascia should be taken in line with skin incision (Fig. 7.2). Just underneath lies the vastus lateralis muscle (Fig. 7.3).

Incision of the fascia in the distal part must be anterior to the lateral intermuscular septum, and then the muscle fibres must be elevated to the septum. Vastus lateralis muscle is retracted anteromedially (Fig. 7.4).

Perforating vessels of the profunda femoris artery and vein should be ligated (Fig. 7.5).

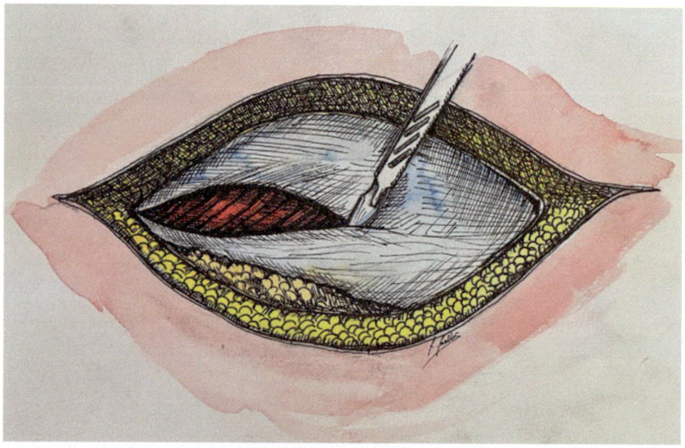

Fig. 7.2 Iliotibial band division.

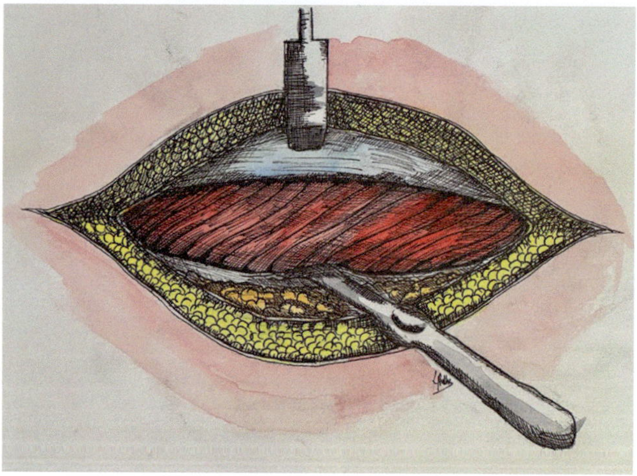

Fig. 7.3 Vastus lateralis muscle is exposed.

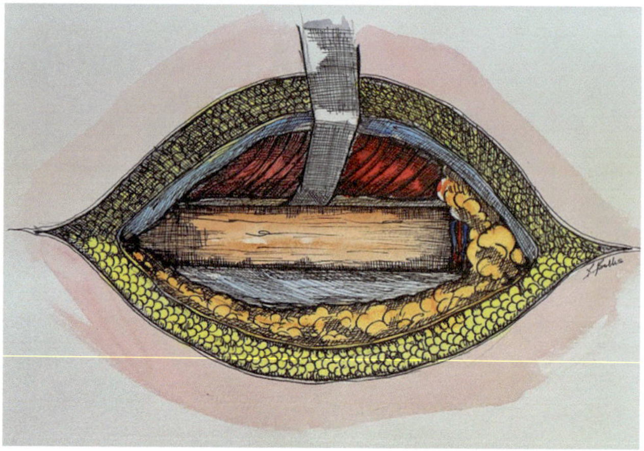

Fig. 7.4 Femur exposition.

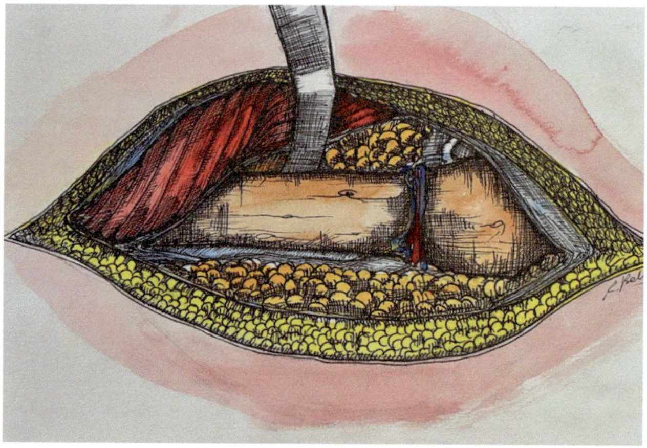

Fig. 7.5 Complete exposition of distal femur.

7.3 Structure at Risk

- No significant structure at risk.
- Peroneal nerve can be damaged (dissection must be anterior to the biceps femoris).

Part II

Knee

8 Anatomy of the Knee

8.1 Introduction

The knee joint is the largest joint of the body, that comprises of articulation between femur and tibia, and femur and patella. The bone shapes, the cruciate ligaments and the ligaments and tendons on the medial and lateral sides of the knee allow six degree of movements, three in translation and three in rotation. Due to complexity of knee, the main approaches are anterior and anterolateral, trying to avoid the tendon structures (patellar and quadriceps tendon) whose section could cause post-operative scar, pain and stiffness. In this chapter the most important anatomical structures will be highlighted by comprehensive drawings and captions.

R. Ballis et al., *Atlas of Orthopaedic Surgical Approaches to the Lower Limbs*, https://doi.org/10.1007/978-3-031-07723-4_8

8.2 Ligaments

8.2.1 Anterior View

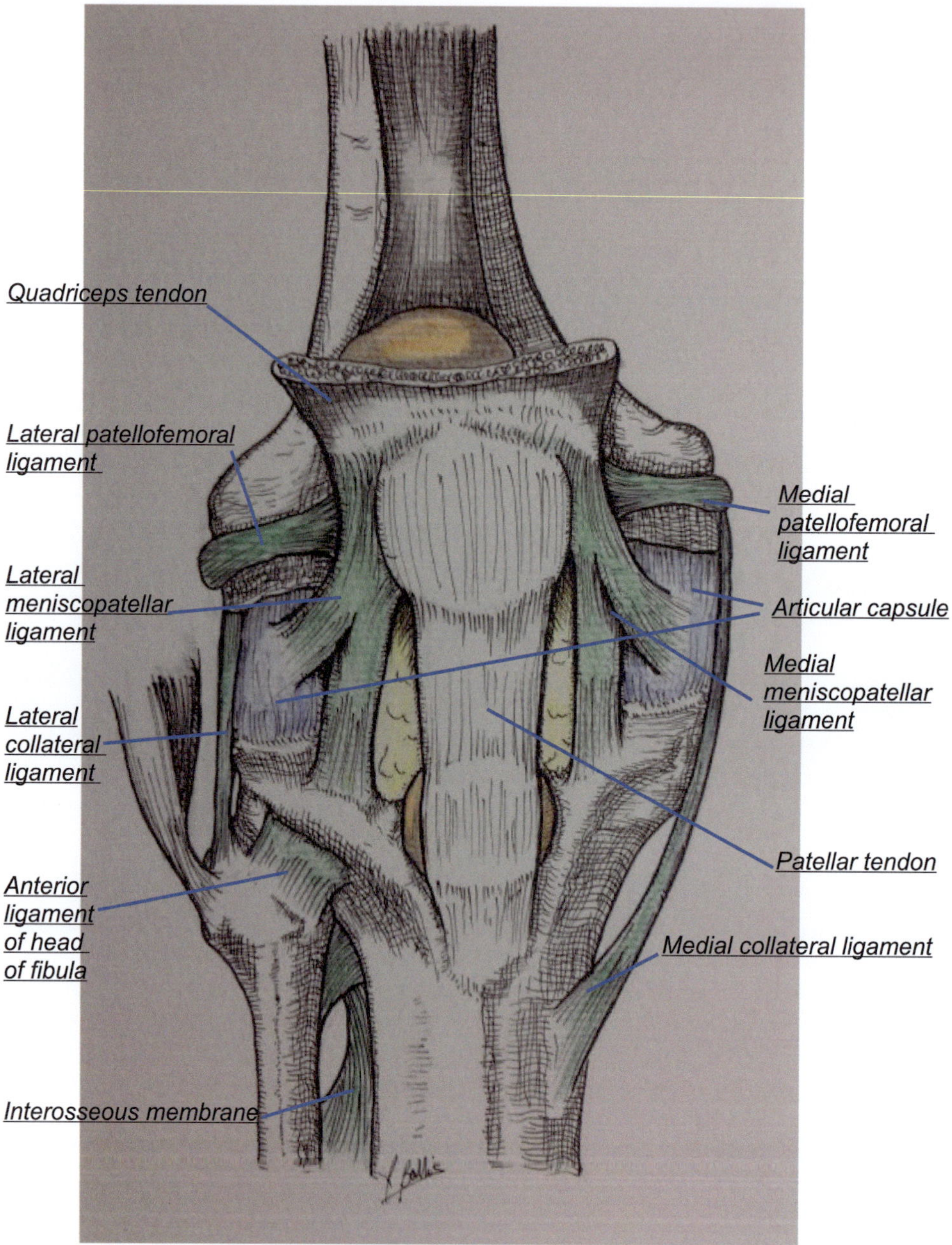

8.2.2 Posterior View

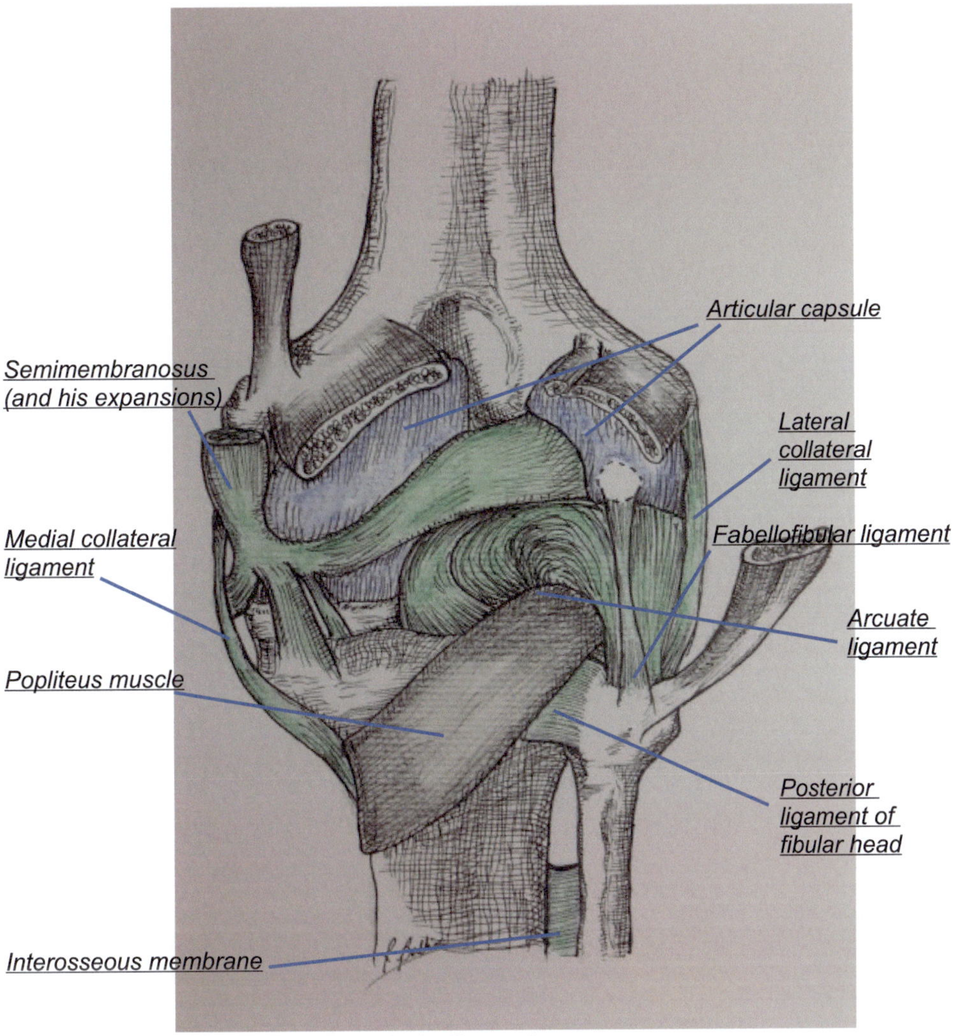

8.3 Nerves

8.3.1 Anterior View

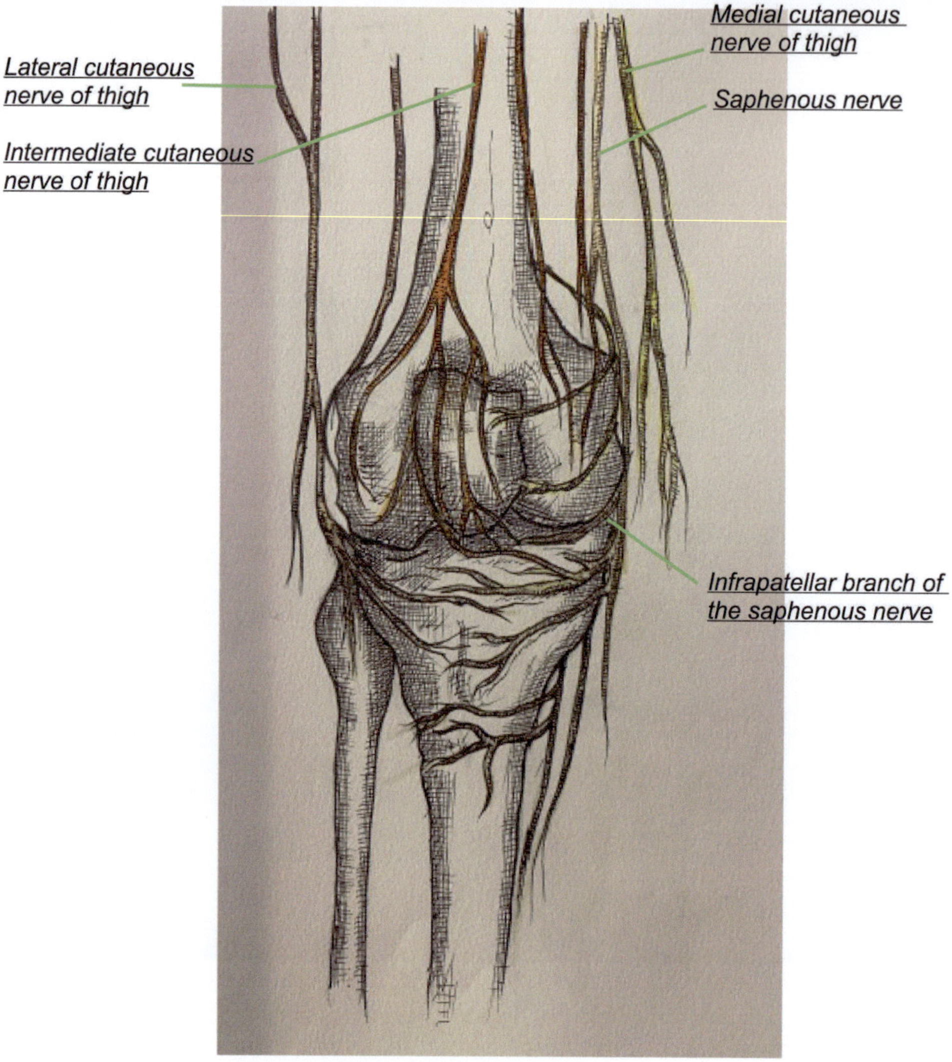

8.3.2 Posterior View

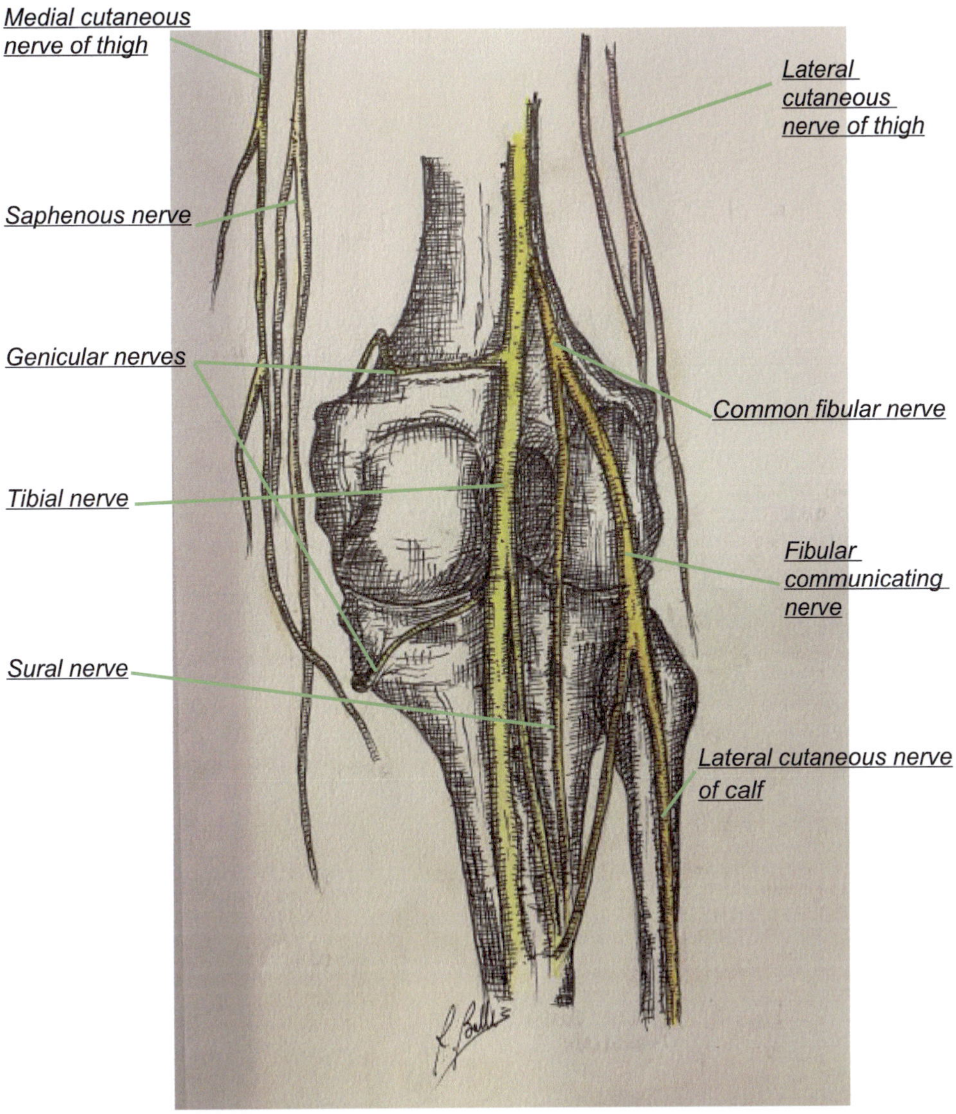

8.4 Arteries

8.4.1 Anterior View

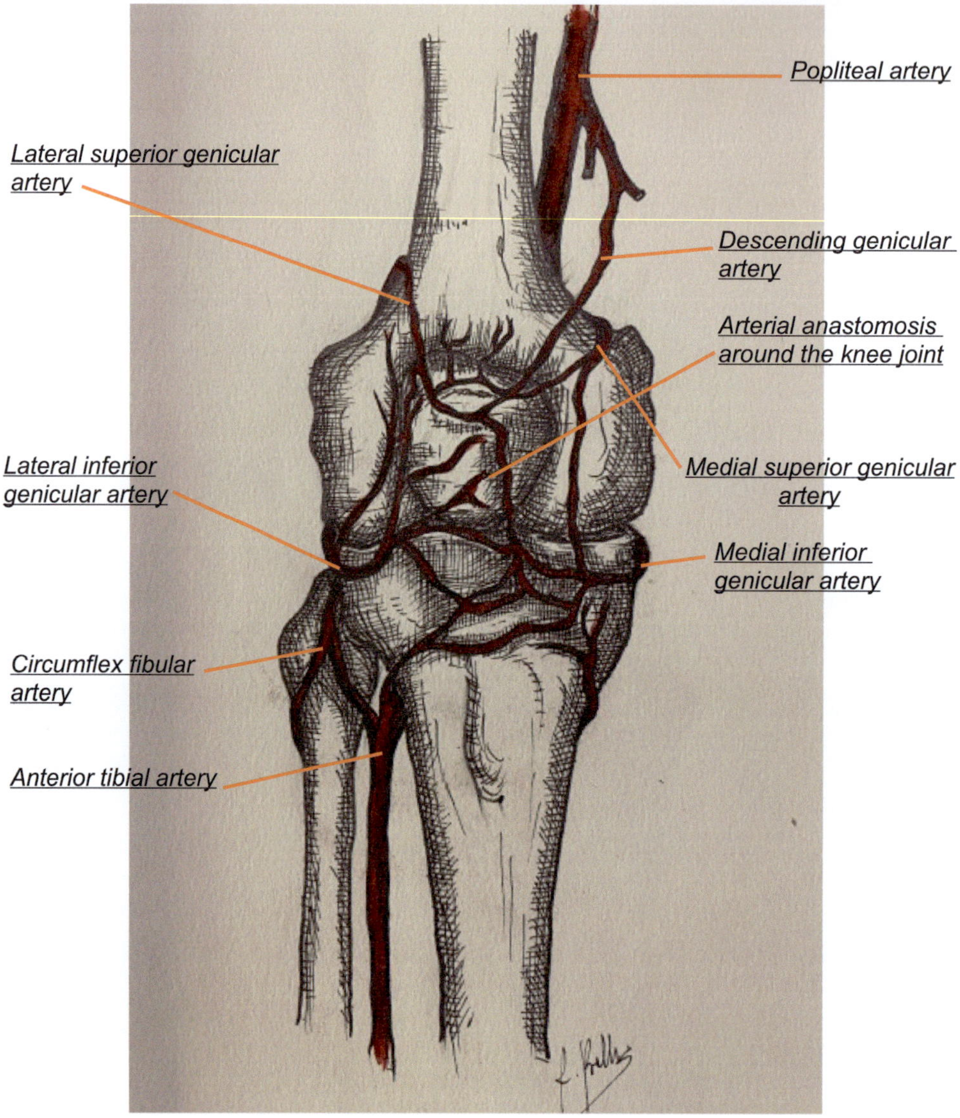

8.4.2 Posterior View

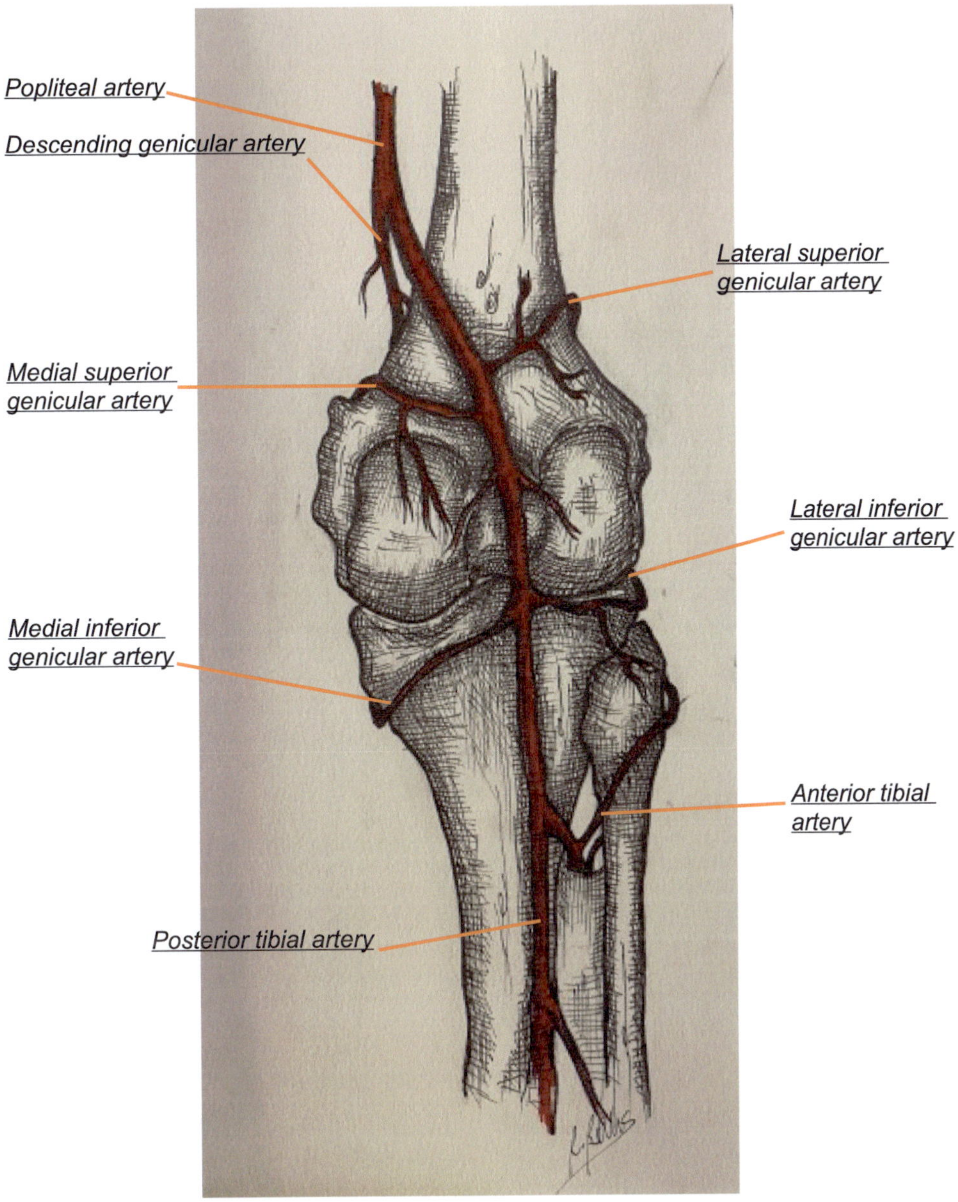

Posterior Approach to the Knee

9

9.1 Introduction

The posterior approach of the knee is less common because the presence of neurovascular structures makes it more challenging. In this chapter the indications, anatomic considerations and tip and tricks and pitfalls of this approach are presented with original drawing images and concise text.

- Indications: Posteromedial tibial plateau fractures, tumors, osteomyelitis, open repair of avulsion fractures of posterior cruciate ligament.
- Position of the patient: The patient should be placed prone. Sterile dressing to allow a free mobilization in flex-extension.
- Landmarks: Fibular head, biceps tendon, posteromedial border of tibia and joint line (identified by flexing and extending the knee).

9.2 Step-by-Step Procedure

– Incision: The incision can be done in S-shaped from proximally lateral to distally medial (Fig. 9.1) or as a L-shaped that starts laterally in the level of popliteal fossa and runs through it and bends distally in the medial edge of gastrocnemius muscle.

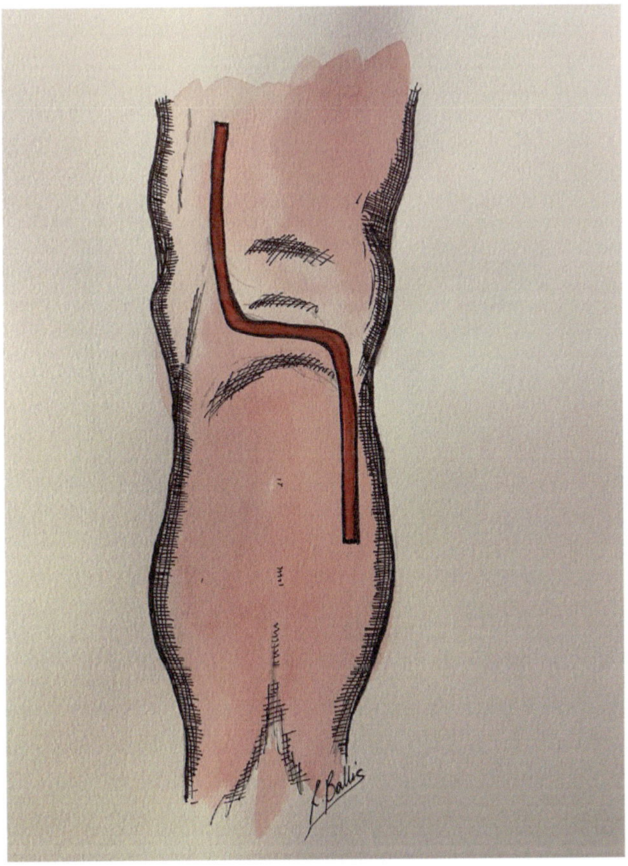

Fig. 9.1 Landmark incision. © Rosa Ballis 2022. All Rights Reserved

R. Ballis et al., *Atlas of Orthopaedic Surgical Approaches to the Lower Limbs*, https://doi.org/10.1007/978-3-031-07723-4_9

- The subcutaneous layer and fascia are dissected in the same direction as the skin incision.
- Identification of the sural nerve (Fig. 9.2) and saphenous vein.
- The popliteal vein and artery stay laterally while the semimembranous muscle medially (Fig. 9.3).
- The plane between the semimembranous muscle and medial head of gastrocnemius must be identified, and a bluntly dissection must be done.

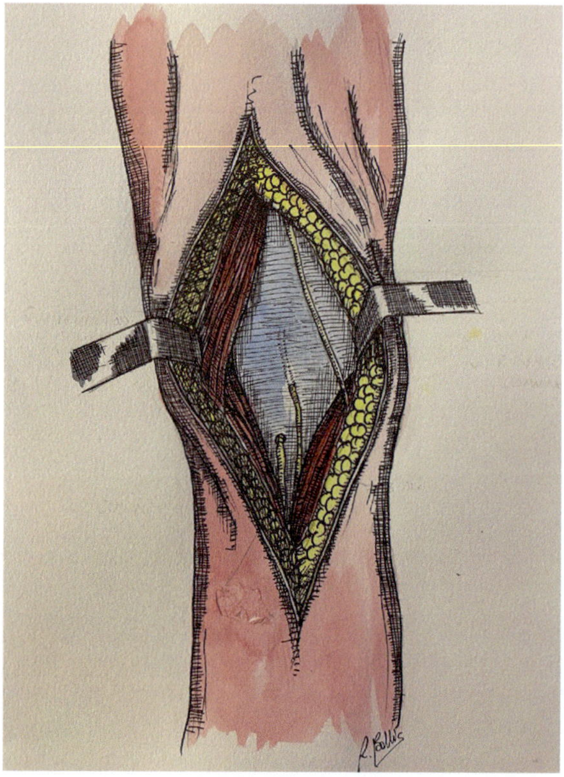

Fig. 9.2 Sural nerve identification.

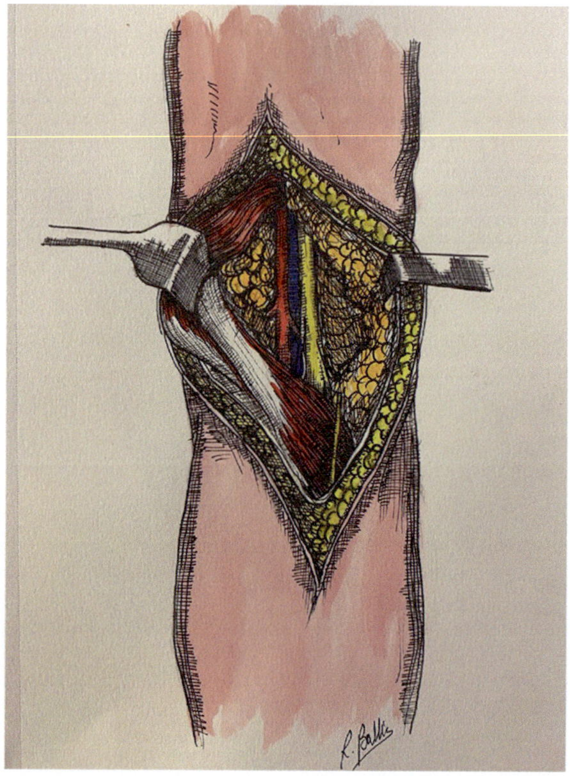

Fig. 9.3 Identification of vasculonervous popliteal complex.

– The anterior edge of gastrocnemius can be transected close to the insertion, and the free muscle is retracted laterally (Fig. 9.4).
– The origin of popliteus muscle is identified. Depending on the planned surgery, the capsule can be dissected and the joint space exposed (Fig. 9.5).

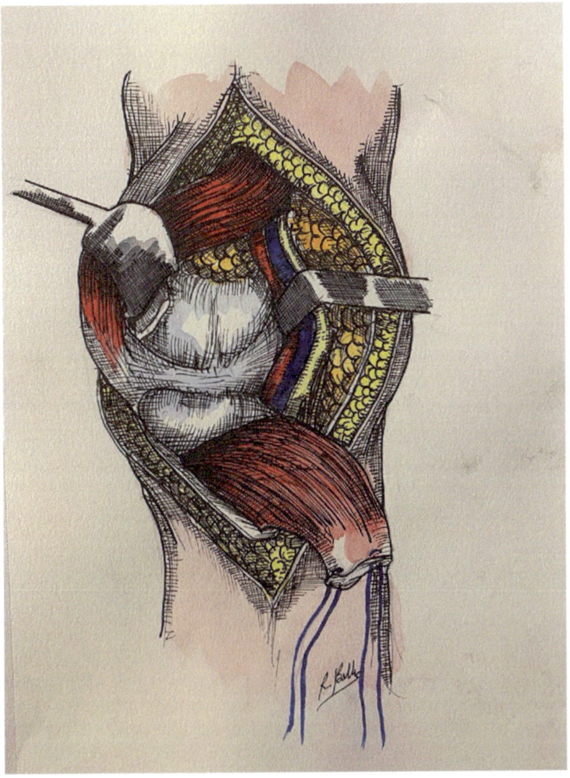

Fig. 9.4 Splitting of the medial head of gastrocnemius muscle.

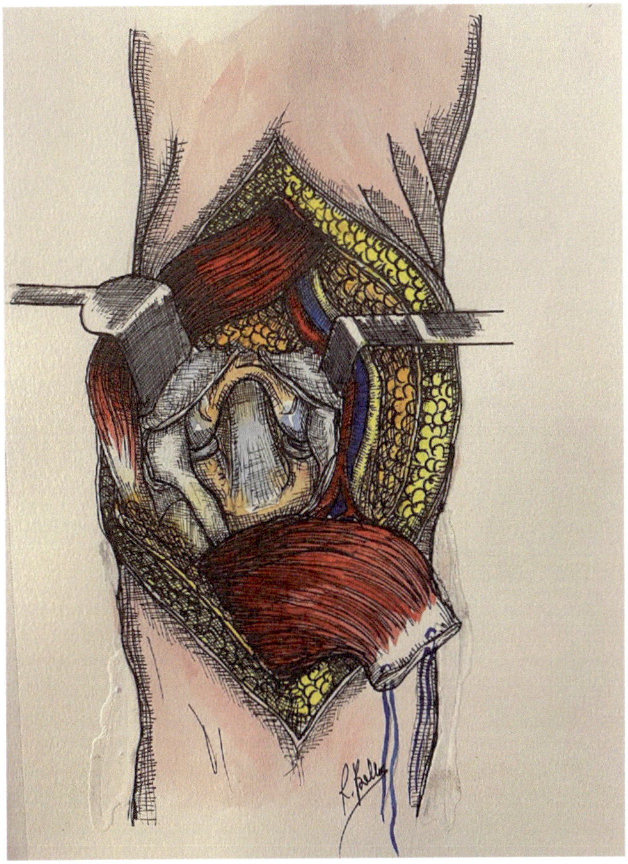

Fig. 9.5 Posterior knee exposed.

9.3 Structures at Risk

- In the first part of dissection, posterior superficial sensitive nerves must be preserved (sural and saphenous).
- Vasculonervous popliteal complex must be identified and protected. It lies laterally.

10 Parapatellar Medial Approach to the Knee

10.1 Introduction

The medial parapatellar approach provides great visualization and extensibility, which made this the most common used approach to the knee. The approach follows the medial border of the quadriceps tendon, and leaves tissue on the patella on which to repair the medial joint capsule.

- Indications: Total knee replacement, unicompartmental medial knee replacement, revision of total/partial knee replacement, medial condyle fracture fixation, distal femoral replacement, synovectomy, patellectomy, knee joint drainage.
- Position of patient: The patient lies supine. If the tourniquet is applied, care should be taken to place it far enough away from the incision. Sterile dressing should be applied allowing free movement of the knee during surgery.
- Landmarks: Tibial tuberosity, patellar tendon, patella, and quadriceps tendon.

10.2 Step-by-Step Procedure

– Incision: Depending on planned surgery, but generally starts 5 cm proximal to the superior pole of patella and straight distally to the proximal third of the tibial tuberosity (Fig. 10.1).

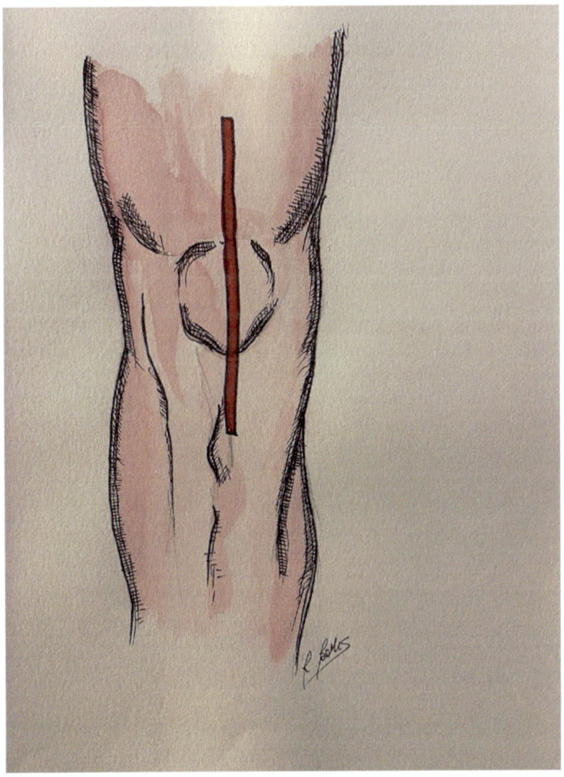

Fig. 10.1 Landmark incision. © Rosa Ballis 2022. All Rights Reserved

R. Ballis et al., *Atlas of Orthopaedic Surgical Approaches to the Lower Limbs*, https://doi.org/10.1007/978-3-031-07723-4_10

- After skin incision, the subcutaneous tissue is divided in line with the incision down to the quadriceps tendon, prepatellar bursa and patellar tendon.
- The prepatellar bursa is then removed (Fig. 10.2).
- Now, the dissection should be done further to the medial retinaculum (Fig. 10.3). Care should be taken to protect infrapatellar branch of saphenous nerve.
- After identifying proximal pole of patella, access to the joint is taken through the quadriceps tendon approximately in the medial third. Care should be taken to leave enough tendon for a good final closure.
- The incision should run distally through the belly of vastus medialis and also here care should be taken to leave enough medial retinaculum for optimal closure.
- The knee joint is finally opened by dissecting the capsule and synovia (Fig. 10.4). The infrapatellar fat pad can be retracted or excised.
- Depending on the planned operation, patella can be subluxated laterally (i.e. medial condyle fracture fixation) or everted (i.e. total knee replacement).

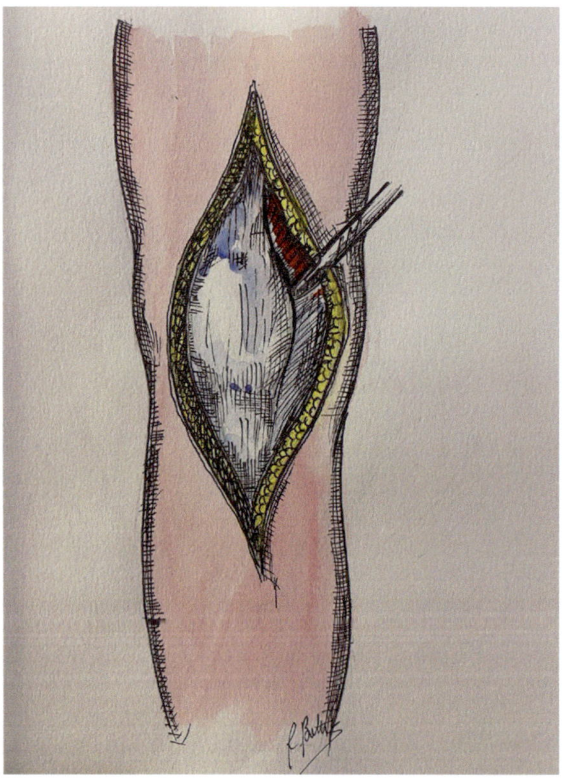

Fig. 10.2 Medial patellar incision. © Rosa Ballis 2022. All Rights Reserved

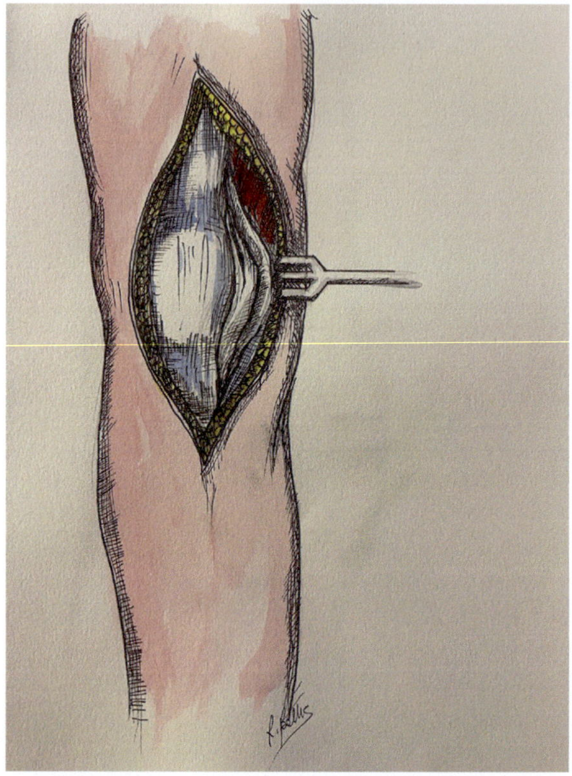

Fig. 10.3 Entering the joint to quadriceps tendon. © Rosa Ballis 2022. All Rights Reserved

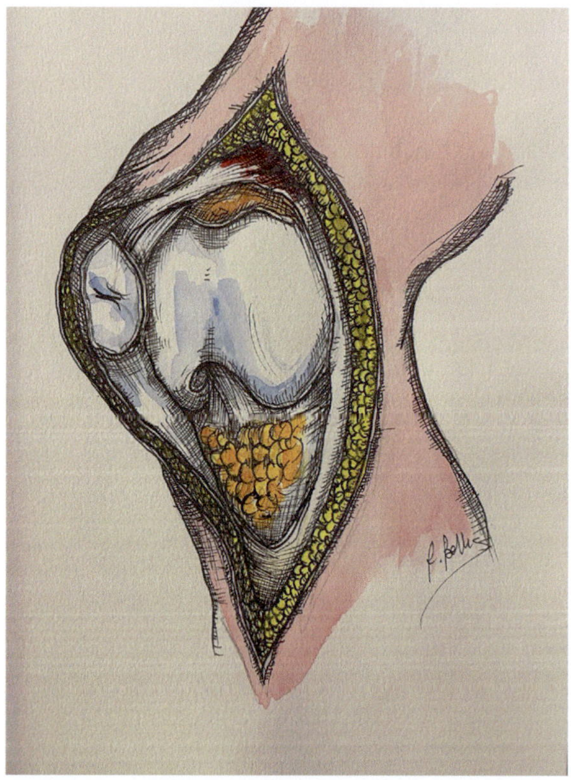

Fig. 10.4 Knee exposure. © Rosa Ballis 2022. All Rights Reserved

10.3 Structures at Risk

- Infrapatellar branch of saphenous nerve.
- Avulsion of patellar ligament from insertion on the tibia should be avoided.
- Anterior insertion of the medial meniscus (unless doing joint replacement).

11 Parapatellar Lateral Approach to the Knee

11.1 Introduction

The lateral parapatellar approach is usually used in pathologies of valgus knee. It provides direct access to the lateral and posterolateral structures, and the possibility to release proper ligament for balancing in total knee replacement.

- Indications: Total knee replacement in severe valgus knee, lateral femoral condyle osteochondritis, lateral meniscectomy, removal of loose bodies.
- Position of the patient: The patient is supine. Depending on the planned operation, a side support is placed and the limb is dressed in flexed position.
- Landmarks: Tibial tuberosity, patellar tendon, patella, quadriceps tendon, head of the fibula and lateral joint line.

11.2 Step-by-Step Procedure

– Incision: Midline above the patella depending on the planned surgery, standard incision starts 5 cm proximal to the upper pole of the patella and continues straight distally to the proximal third of the pole of the tibial tuberosity (Fig. 11.1).

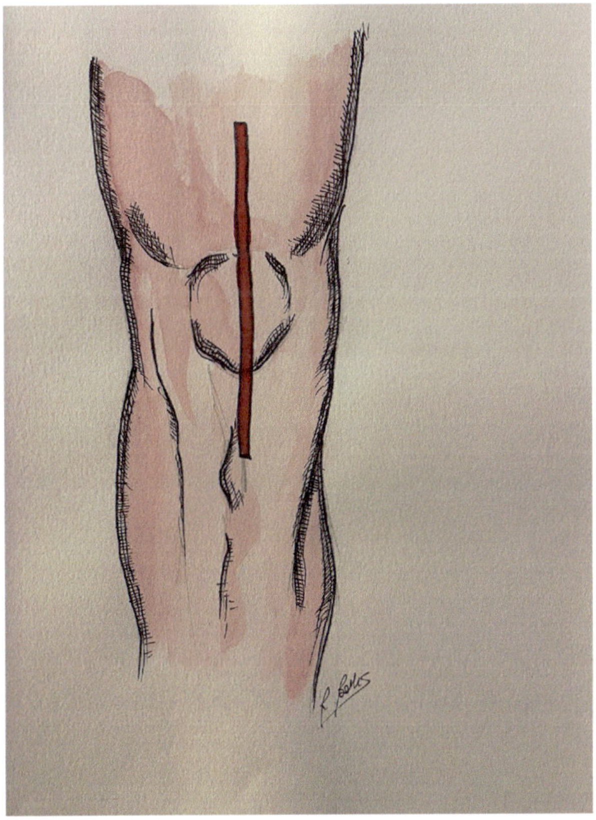

Fig. 11.1 Landmark incision. © Rosa Ballis 2022. All Rights Reserved

R. Ballis et al., *Atlas of Orthopaedic Surgical Approaches to the Lower Limbs*, https://doi.org/10.1007/978-3-031-07723-4_11

- Exposure is the same as in medial parapatellar approach (Fig. 11.2).
- Arthrotomy is carried in the lateral side of patella leaving 2 mm tendon left for closure (Fig. 11.3).
- Knee joint is exposed and Hoffa's fat pad is bluntly pushed off the lateral retinaculum, so it can be used later as an additional augmentation (Fig. 11.4).

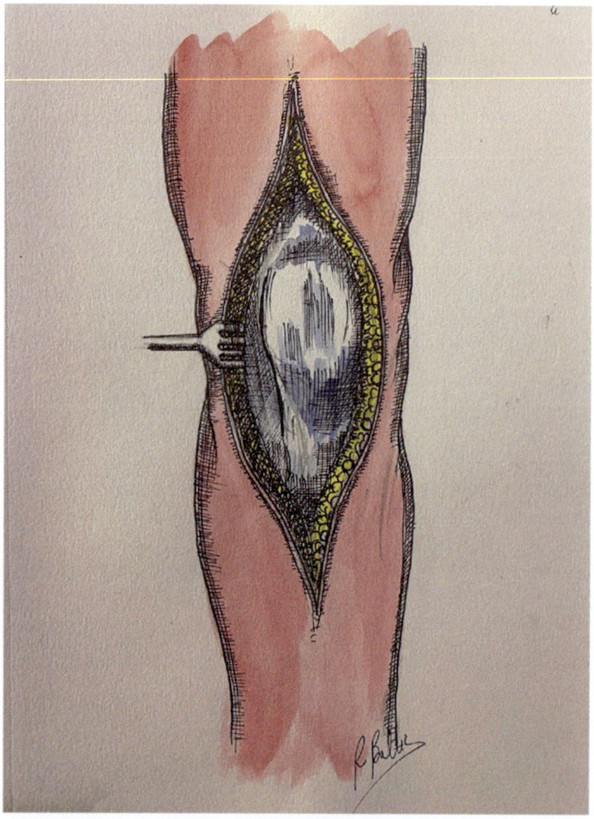

Fig. 11.2 Lateral parapatellar incision. © Rosa Ballis 2022. All Rights Reserved

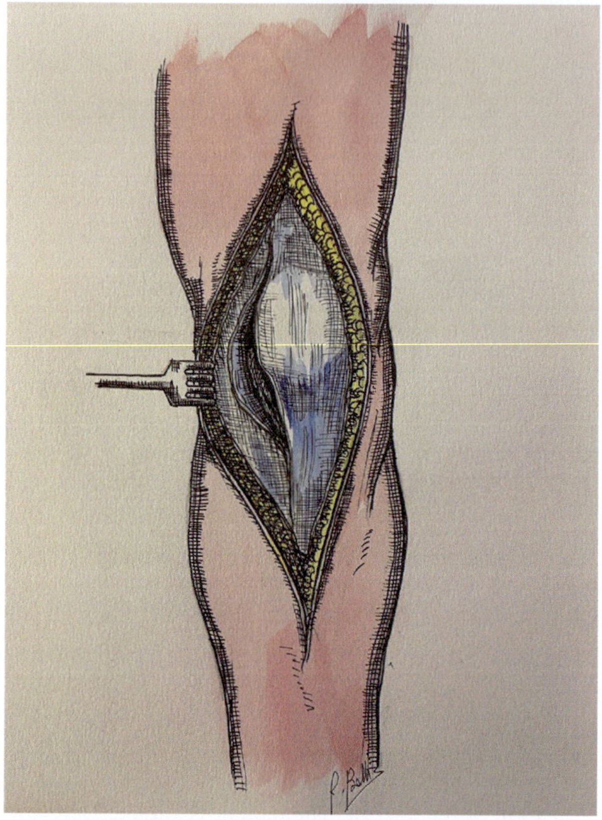

Fig. 11.3 Arthrotomy. © Rosa Ballis 2022. All Rights Reserved

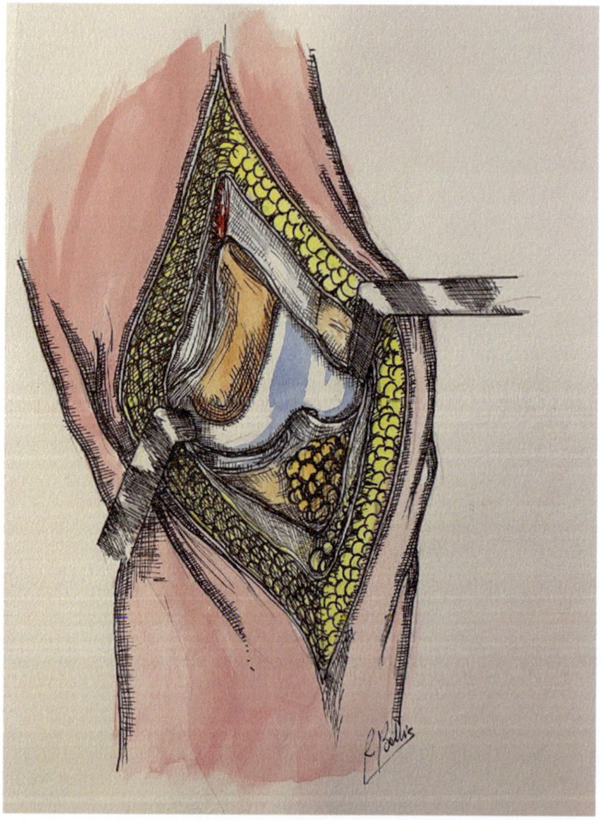

Fig. 11.4 Lateral knee exposure. © Rosa Ballis 2022. All Rights Reserved

11.3 Structures at Risk

- Lateral inferior genicular artery: It can cause massive postoperative hemarthrosis.
- Fibular collateral ligament (LCL).
- Lateral meniscus attachment.

12 Hamstring Harvest

12.1 Introduction

Hamstring tendon is the most commonly used autograft for anterior cruciate ligament reconstruction. It has relatively low site morbidity and the technique is straightforward. Besides ACL reconstruction, the hamstring graft has been used in other ligament and tendon reconstructions and repairs in shoulder, ankle and knee.

- Indications: Graft for: Anterior Cruciate ligament (ACL) reconstruction; Medial patello-femoral ligament reconstruction, acromio-clavicular ligament reconstruction, coraco-clavicular ligament reconstruction etc. The pes anserinus has close relationships with the saphenous nerve and its relative branches, in particular the infrapatellar one (Fig. 12.1).
- Position of the patient: The patient lies in supine position. The leg is positioned knee flexed 90° with possibility of extension.
- Landmarks: Tibial tubercle and medial border of tibia.

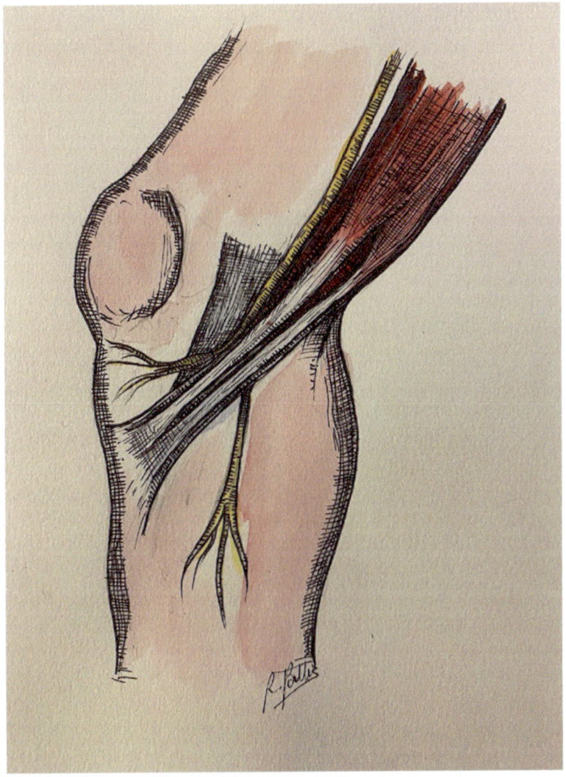

Fig. 12.1 Anatomy of pes anserinus. © Rosa Ballis 2022. All Rights Reserved

R. Ballis et al., *Atlas of Orthopaedic Surgical Approaches to the Lower Limbs*, https://doi.org/10.1007/978-3-031-07723-4_12

12.2 Step-by-Step Procedure

- Incision: Is horizontal or oblique and starts proximally from the line between tibial tubercle and medial border of tibia advancing 1.5–2 cm distally (Fig. 12.2).
- Dissection of the superficial tissue is made in line with the incision and after exposure of the sartorial fascia (Fig. 12.3).
- Fascia is incised and insertion of hamstrings is exposed.
- Gracilis tendon which lies more superficially is taken with a Kelly forceps and mobilized.
- Semitendinosus is now identified and grabbed with another forceps (Fig. 12.4).
- Tension bands are released, especially in the semitendinosus tendon before introducing the stripper.
- Harvest may be started releasing the tendons from the insertions or not.

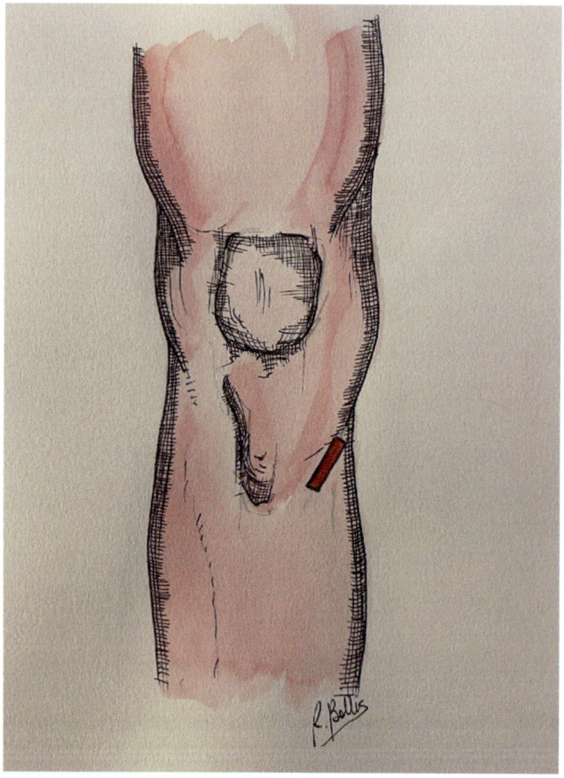

Fig. 12.2 Landmark incision. © Rosa Ballis 2022. All Rights Reserved

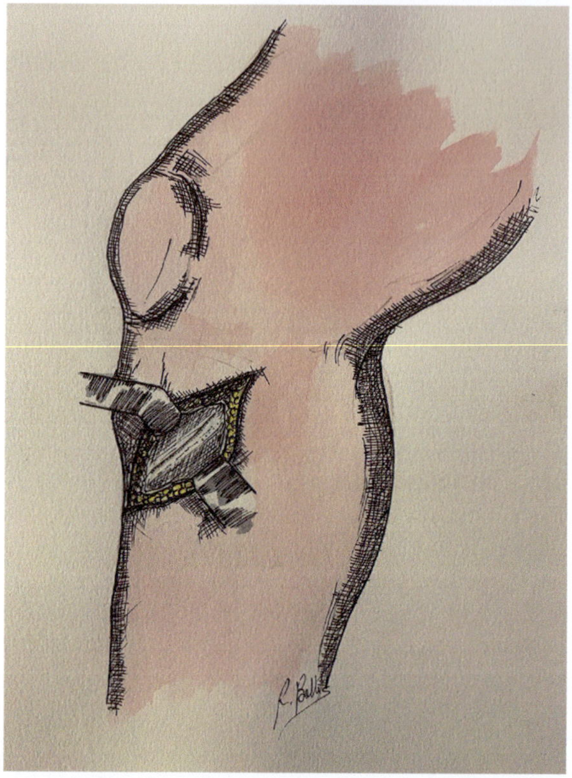

Fig. 12.3 Sartorial fascia. © Rosa Ballis 2022. All Rights Reserved

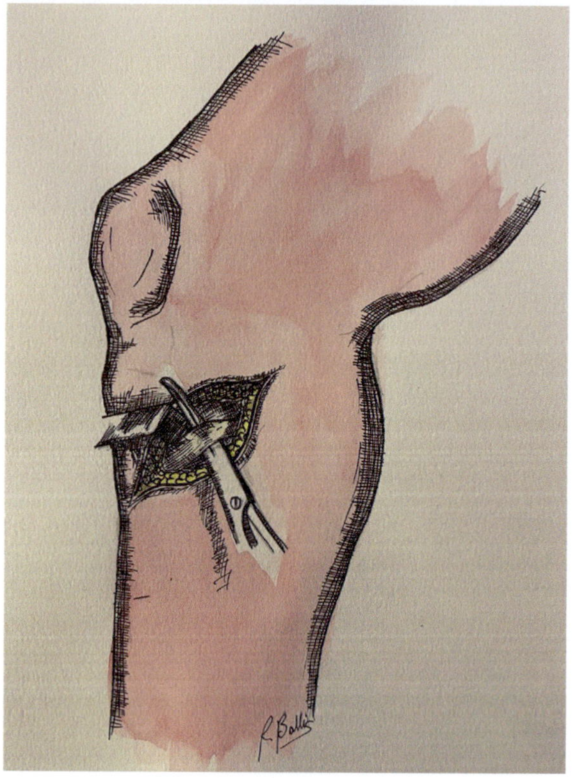

Fig. 12.4 Gracilis tendon. © Rosa Ballis 2022. All Rights Reserved

– Tendon is grasped pushing firmly the stripper (Fig. 12.5). If a stoppage is perceived and it is impossible to move the stripper, it must be removed and made another check that there are no tension bands, otherwise the graft can be cut.

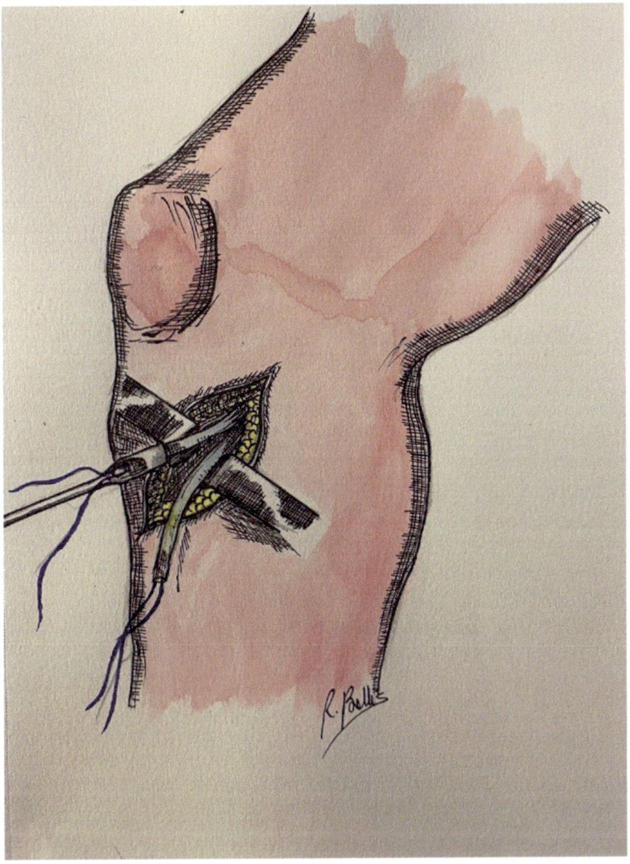

Fig. 12.5 Hamstring harvest with tendon stripper. © Rosa Ballis 2022. All Rights Reserved

12.3 Structures at Risk

- Infrapatellar branch of the saphenous nerve during tendon dissection. It lies behind them.

Posteromedial Proximal Approach to the Tibia

13

13.1 Introduction

The posteromedial approach to proximal tibial is usually performed in typical shear fractures of the tibial plateau.

- Indications: Medial and complex bicondylar tibial plateau fractures, osteomyelitis, tumour biopsy.
- Position of the patient: The patient is positioned supine. The leg in covered with sterile drapes so it can be moved freely. A sandbag can be placed in the contralateral hip so the external rotation of leg can be increased.
- Landmarks: Tibial tuberosity, joint line, posteromedial surface of tibia.

13.2 Step-by-Step Procedure

– Incision: Skin incision is performed just behind the posteromedial edge of the tibial plateau. The length is determined by planned surgery (Fig 13.1).
– During dissection of subcutaneous layers, attention should be paid to saphenous vein and nerve which pass anterior to the approach.

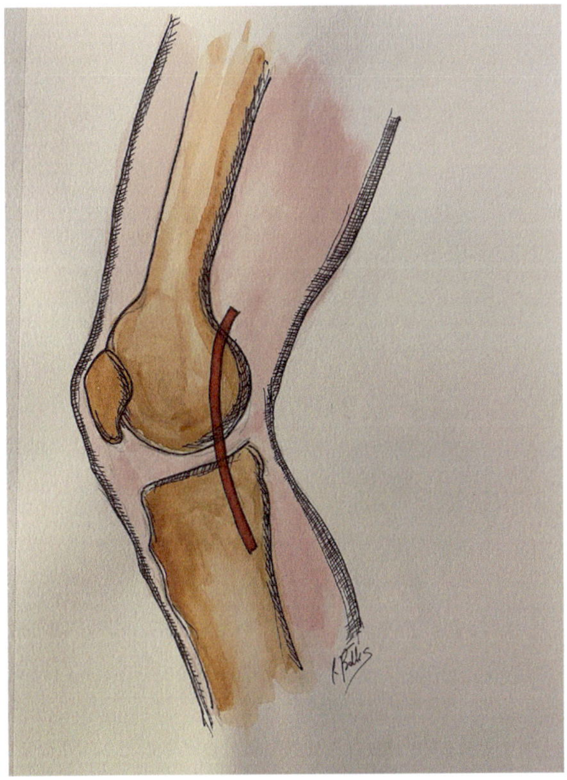

Fig. 13.1 Incision landmark. © Rosa Ballis 2022. All Rights Reserved

R. Ballis et al., *Atlas of Orthopaedic Surgical Approaches to the Lower Limbs*, https://doi.org/10.1007/978-3-031-07723-4_13

- After opening the underlying fascia, the anterior border of pes anserinus is identified (Fig. 13.2), and all three tendons are reflected posteriorly (Fig. 13.3).
- The tendons are resected partially from tibial insertion in order to facilitate the approach.
- Now the posteromedial border of tibia is exposed and the medial head of gastrocnemius and soleus muscle can be seen.
- Then, in line with the approach, the capsule and synovia can be dissected and the joint space exposed (Fig. 13.4).

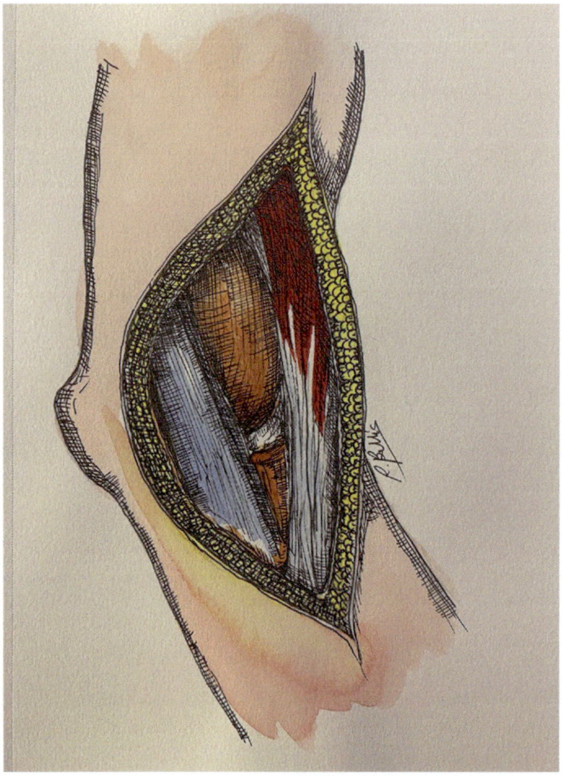

Fig. 13.2 Exposition of pes anserinus.

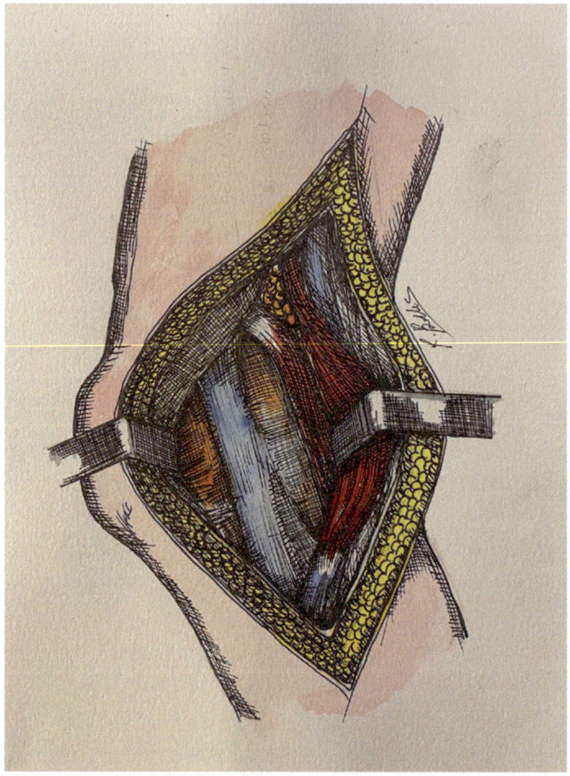

Fig. 13.3 Retraction of pes anserinus.

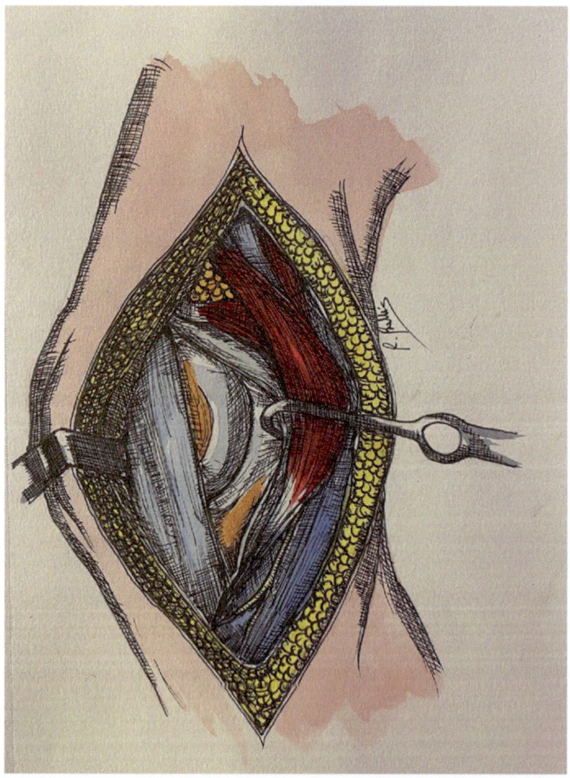

Fig. 13.4 Exposition of the posteomedial edge of tibia.

13.3 Structures at Risk

- Care must be taken to not damage the nutrient artery at the level of the middle of the tibial shaft (important for the blood supply); for this reason, complete dissection of the periosteum at the interosseous margin should not be carried out.

14 Lateral Proximal Approach to the Tibia

14.1 Introduction

The lateral approach is mainly used for addressing the lateral tibial plateau fractures. It is a safe and direct approach to the pathological zone.

- Indications: Lateral tibial fractures, osteomyelitis, tumour biopsy, bone graft harvest.
- Position of the patient: The patient is supine. A sandbag is placed under the ipsilateral thigh in order to neutralize the external rotation of the leg. A posterior support can be added in order to keep the knee flexed.
- Landmarks: Tibial shaft, anterior tibial margin, Gerdy's tubercle, knee lateral joint line.

14.2 Step-by-Step Procedure

- Incision: Starts at the level of lateral femoral condyle and can be oblique or inverted L-shaped. The incision should continue lateral to the border of the patella and patellar tendon, over Gerdy's tubercle and distally parallel to the anterior tibial border around 1 cm (Fig. 14.1). The length is chosen by surgeon preference.
- The subcutaneous fat is dissected, and the fascia and the iliotibial band (ITB) are exposed.

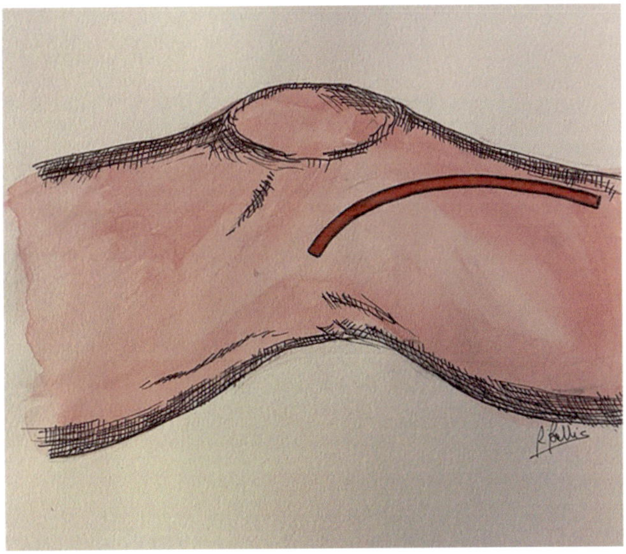

Fig. 14.1 Landmark incision. © Rosa Ballis 2022. All Rights Reserved

R. Ballis et al., *Atlas of Orthopaedic Surgical Approaches to the Lower Limbs*, https://doi.org/10.1007/978-3-031-07723-4_14

- The ITB is splitted from proximal to distal in line with the direction of the fibres running to Gerdy's tubercle (Fig. 14.2).
- Distally and lower leg fascia is incised.
- The tibialis anterior muscle is detached from tibia with a rasp, and ITB is dissected on the Gerdy's tubercle.
- Dissection is usually preferred in the plane between periosteum and muscle (Fig. 14.3).

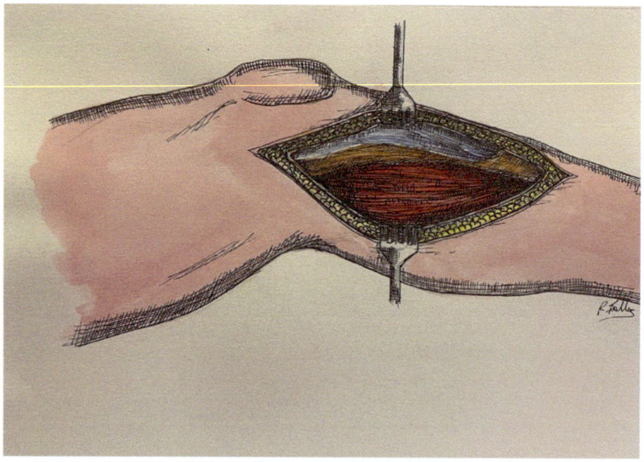

Fig. 14.2 The subcutaneous plane. © Rosa Ballis 2022. All Rights Reserved

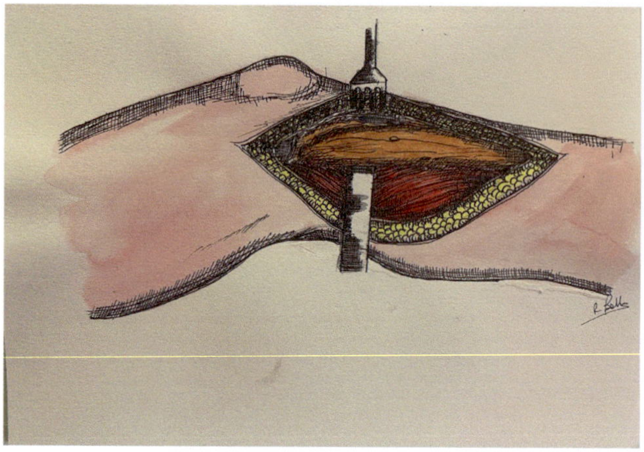

Fig. 14.3 Detachment of tibialis anterior muscle. © Rosa Ballis 2022. All Rights Reserved

14.3 Structures at Risk

- Peroneal nerve (lies posteriorly)
- Lateral meniscus (it must not be completely detached)
- Popliteal vessels (protected by flexing the joint)

Part III

Tibia and Fibula

Anatomy of the Leg

15

15.1 Introduction

Leg is the region between knee and ankle and it is an important structure in weightbearing and movement. Leg comprises of two bones and three muscle compartments. Knowledge of the anatomy of this region is essential in order to make the right surgical approaches to avoid damage of neurovascular structures and skin.

R. Ballis et al., *Atlas of Orthopaedic Surgical Approaches to the Lower Limbs*, https://doi.org/10.1007/978-3-031-07723-4_15

15.2 Muscles

15.2.1 Anterior View

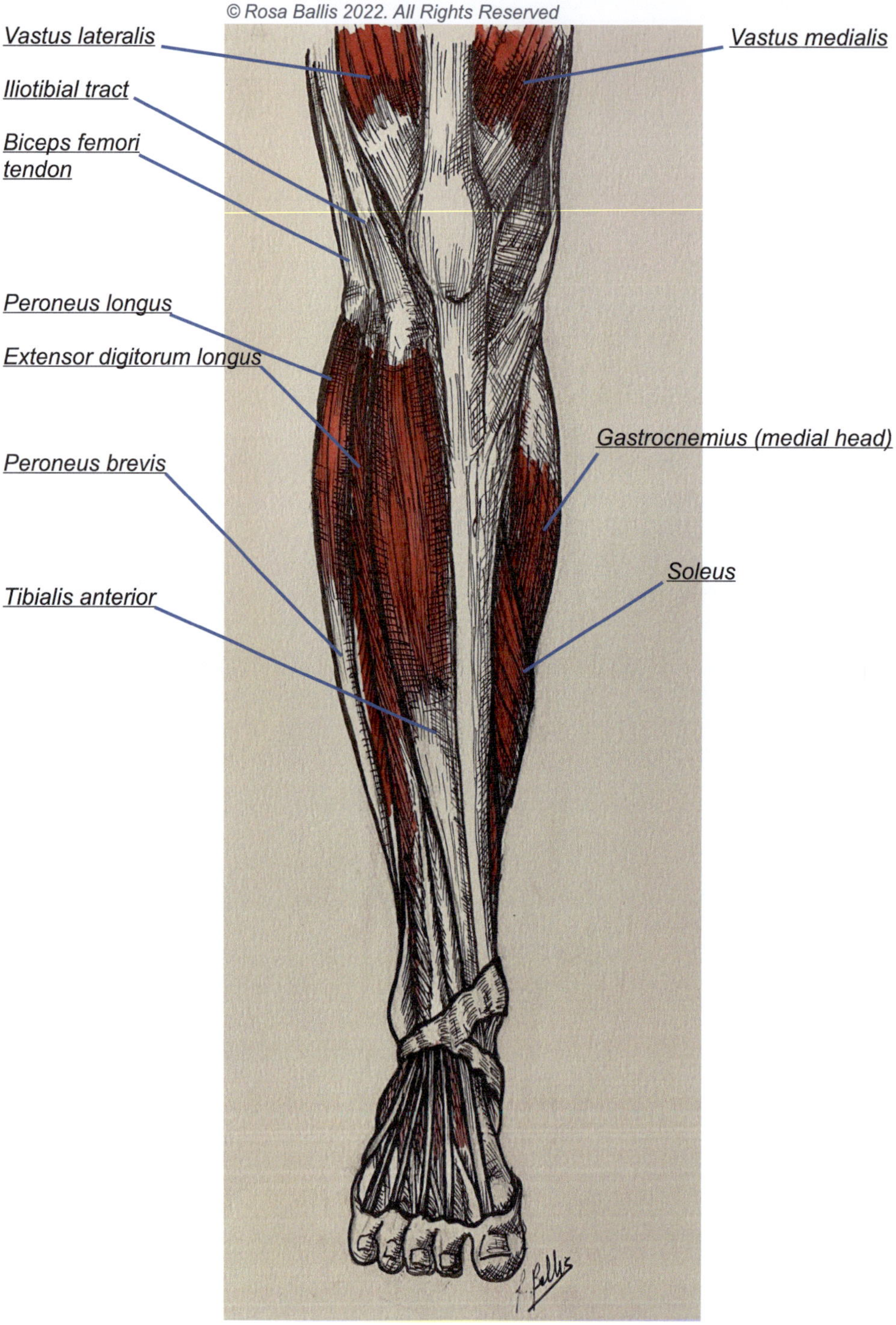

15.2.2 Lateral View

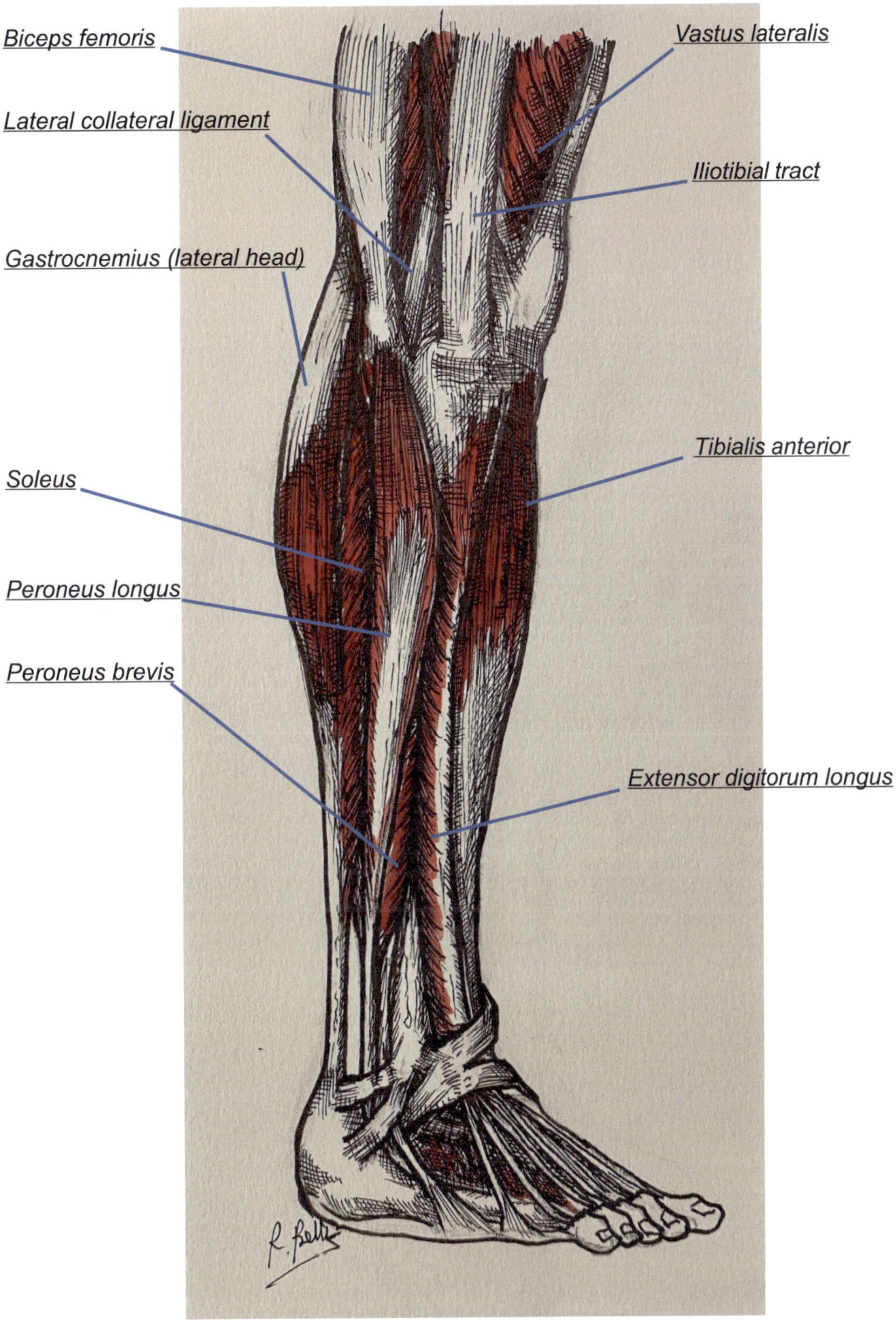

15.2.3 Medial View

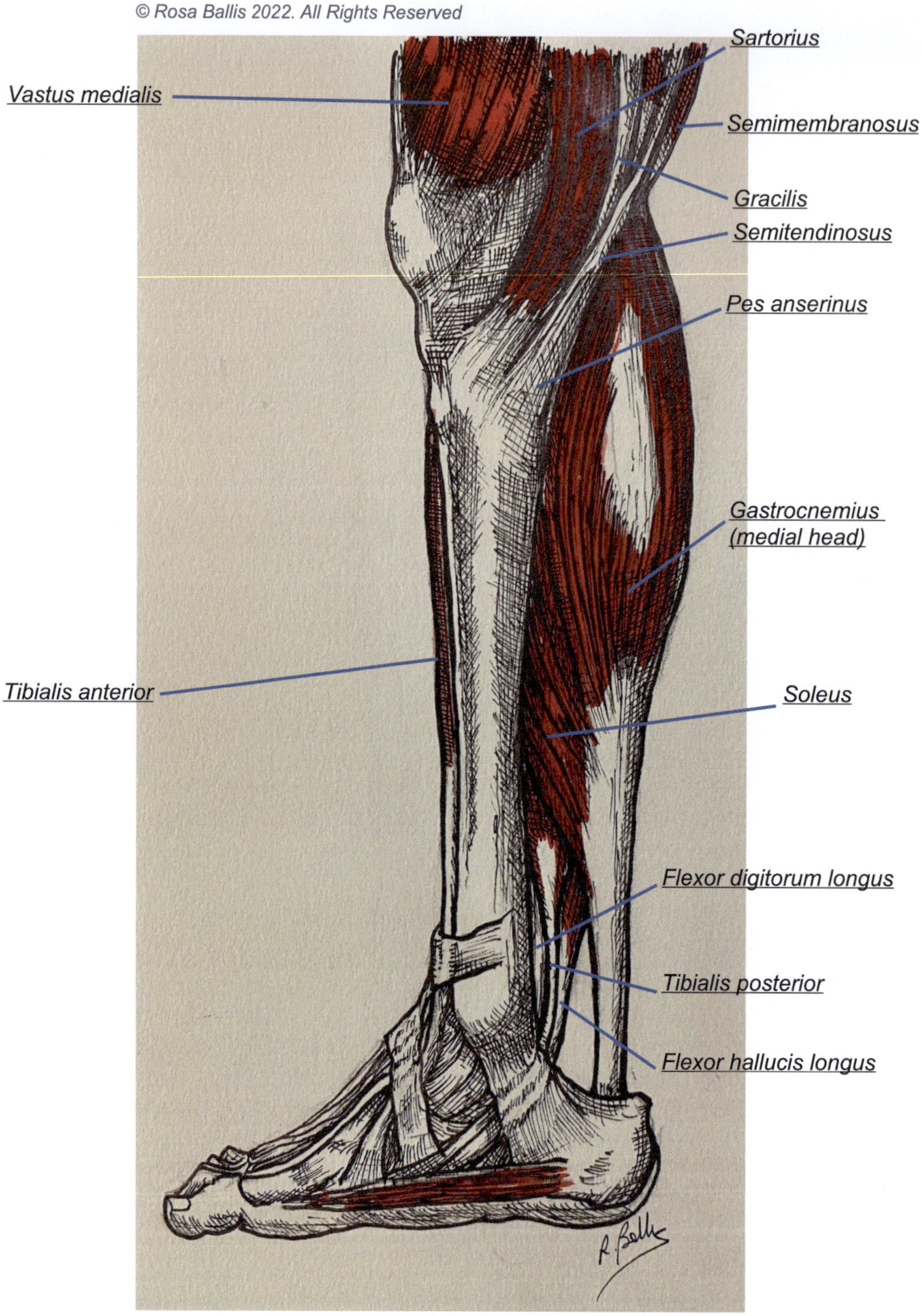

15.2.4 Posterior View

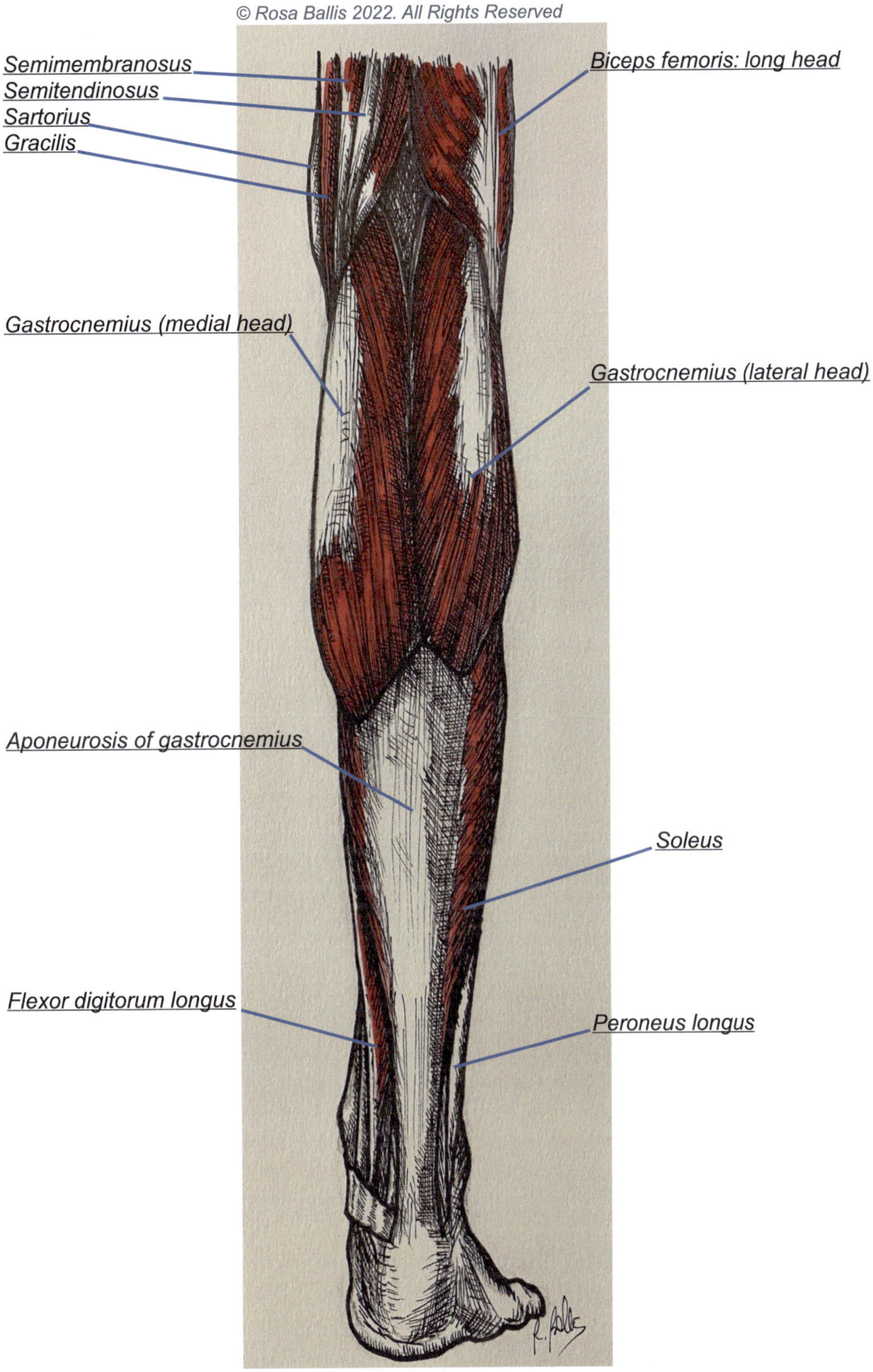

15.3 Nerves

15.3.1 Anterior View

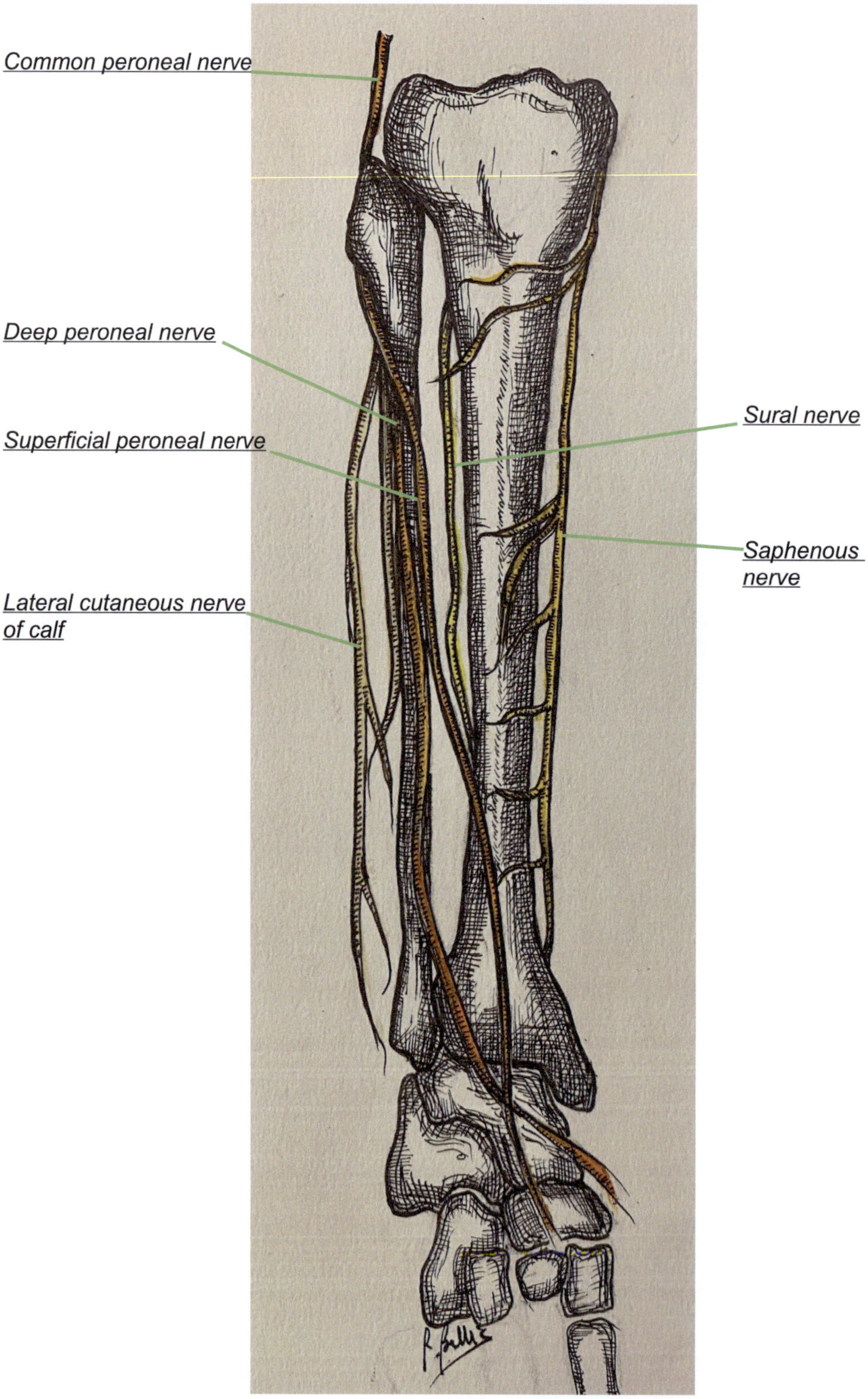

15.3.2 Posterior View

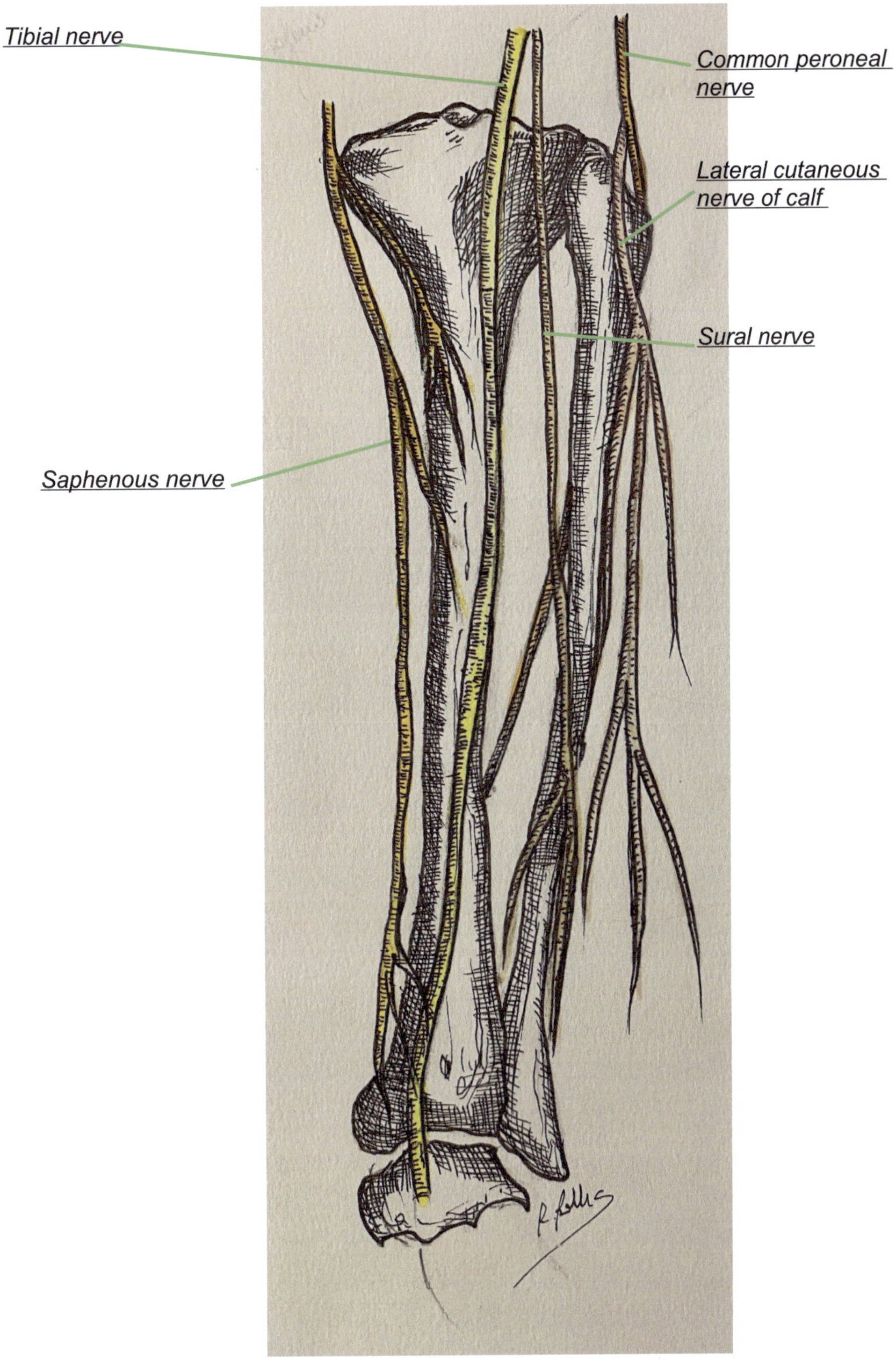

15.4 Arteries

15.4.1 Anterior view

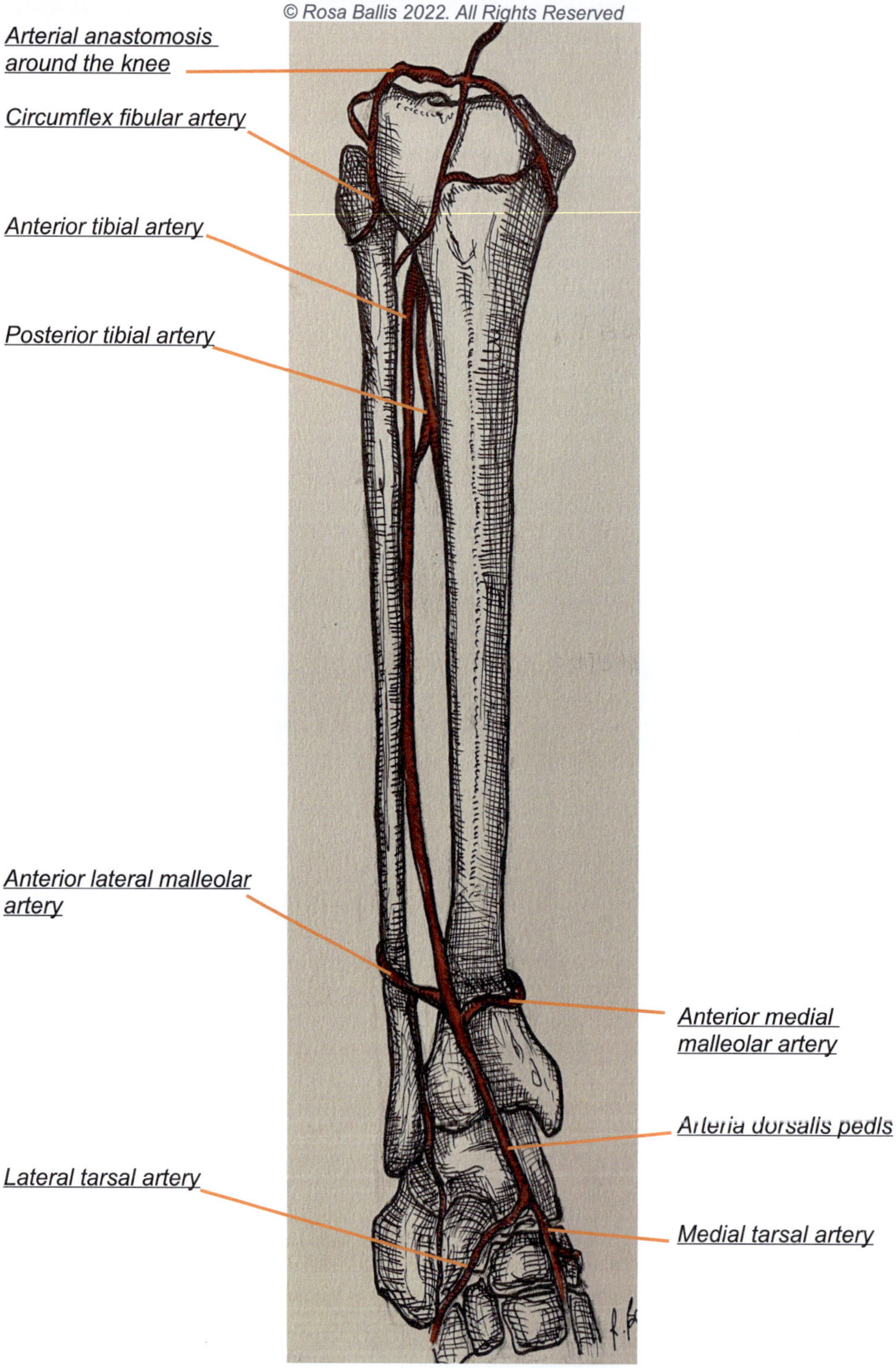

15.4.2 Posterior view

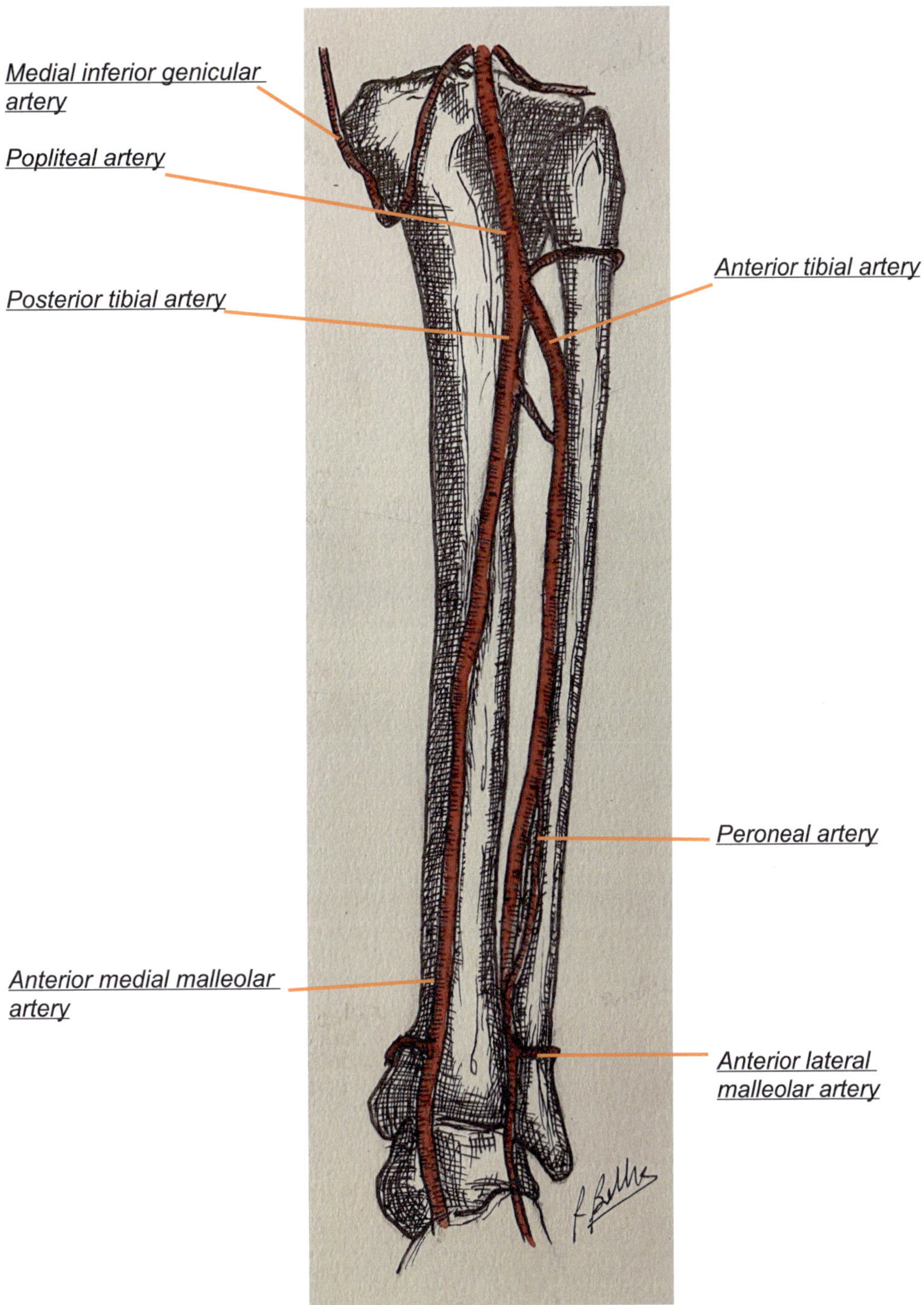

16 Anteromedial Approach to the Leg

16.1 Introduction

Anteromedial approach in the tibia is mostly used for the distal part. It provides great visualization of the medial malleoli and medial and central articular area. Care must be taken to prevent skin necrosis.

- Indications: Fractures of the mid-distal tibia, distal tibial osteotomy, tumour biopsy, osteomyelitis.
- Position of the patient: Usually the patients lie in supine position.
- Landmarks: End of the triangular tibia and posteromedial surface of tibia.

16.2 Step-by-Step Procedure

– Incision: Skin incision begins in the posteromedial border of tibia. The length depends on the procedure (Fig. 16.1).

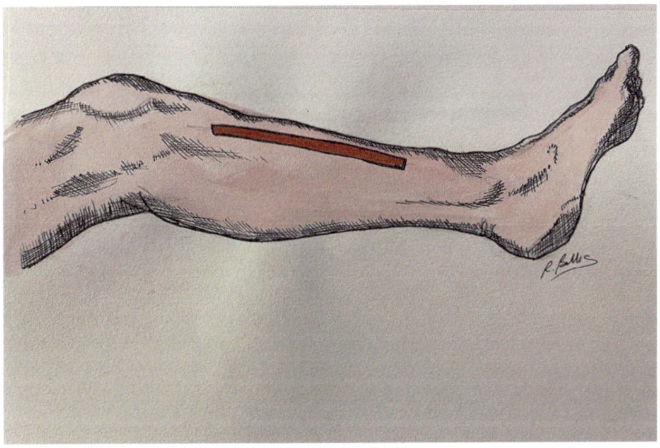

Fig. 16.1 Landmark incision.

R. Ballis et al., *Atlas of Orthopaedic Surgical Approaches to the Lower Limbs*, https://doi.org/10.1007/978-3-031-07723-4_16

- After skin incision and subcutaneous dissection, there is immediately the posteromedial surface of tibia.
- The medial head of gastrocnemius and soleus can be elevated posteriorly by blunt dissection (Figs. 16.2 and 16.3).

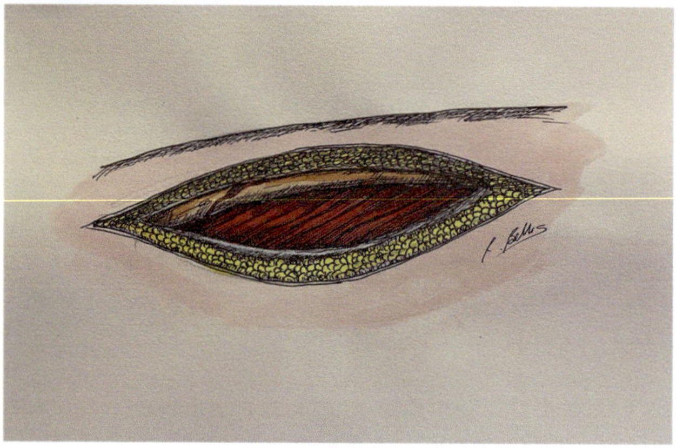

Fig. 16.2 Soleus muscle © Rosa Ballis 2022. All Rights Reserved

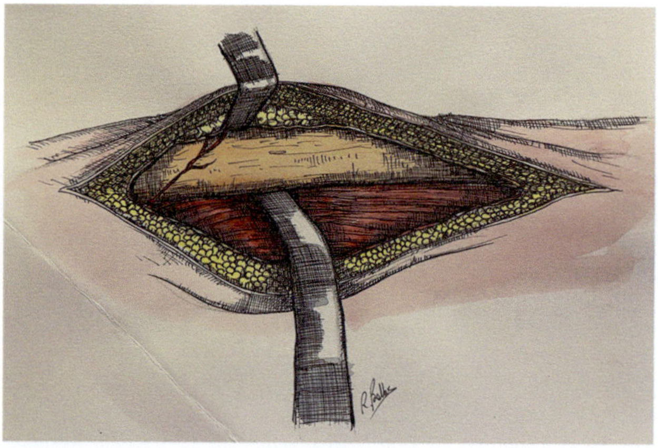

Fig. 16.3 Tibia exposition © Rosa Ballis 2022. All Rights Reserved

16.3 Structures at Risk

- Due to the importance of soft tissue vascularization, the bone exposure should be limited to a minimum.
- Protecting saphenous nerve and vein in the inferior part of the incision is mandatory.

Anterolateral Distal Approach to the Leg

17

17.1 Introduction

The anterolateral approach of the distal tibia offers access at tibial articular surface and fibula, while providing good soft tissue cover. In this chapter, we describe with text and images the anterolateral distal approach to the leg, tips and tricks and pitfalls.

- Indications: Pilon fractures, osteomyelitis, tumours
- Position of the patient: Usually the patient lies in supine position.
- Landmarks: Distal fibula, anterior edge of tibia, fourth metatarsal.

17.2 Step-by-Step Procedure

– Incision: The skin incision begins proximally in the direction of the ankle joint, parallel to the fourth metatarsal and between tibia and fibula (Fig. 17.1).

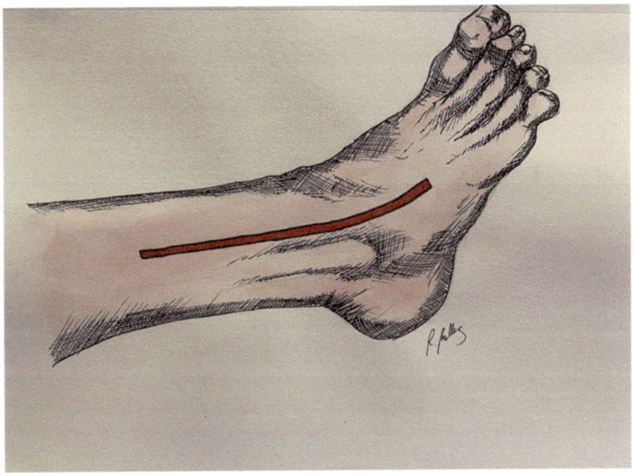

Fig. 17.1 Landmarks incision. © Rosa Ballis 2022. All Rights Reserved

R. Ballis et al., *Atlas of Orthopaedic Surgical Approaches to the Lower Limbs*, https://doi.org/10.1007/978-3-031-07723-4_17

- The fascia of the anterior compartment is dissected (Fig. 17.2).
- The anterior compartment is retracted medially including the extensor digitorum communis longus, the superficial peroneal nerve and the vasculonervous complex: anterior tibial artery, anterior tibial nerve.
- The extensor digitorum communis longus and the peroneus anterior are detached from the anteromedial surface of the fibula.
- The anastomosis between lateral malleolar artery and branch of the peroneal artery must be coagulated (Fig. 17.3).
- Underneath lie the anterior compartment muscles, ligaments and joint capsule.
- The fascia of the extensor digitorum brevis may be incised and retracted medially and the talar neck is exposed (Fig. 17.4).

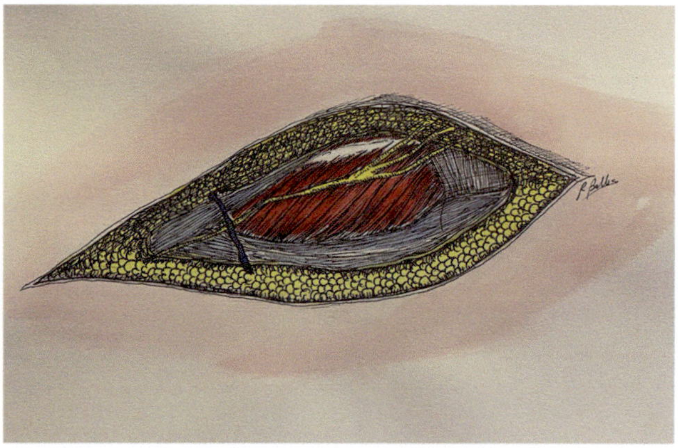

Fig. 17.2 Superficial peroneal nerve. © Rosa Ballis 2022. All Rights Reserved

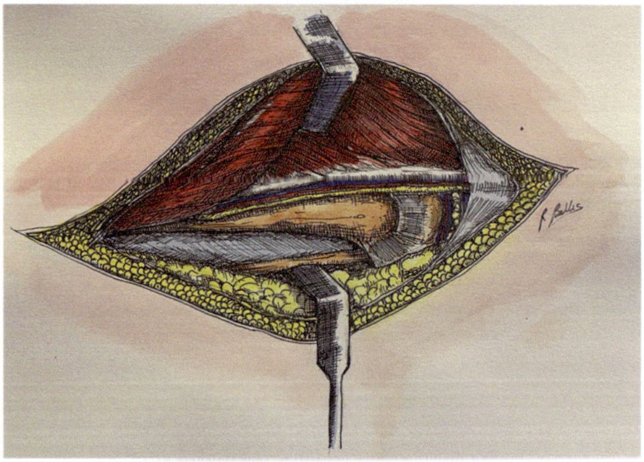

Fig. 17.3 Deep dissection. © Rosa Ballis 2022. All Rights Reserved

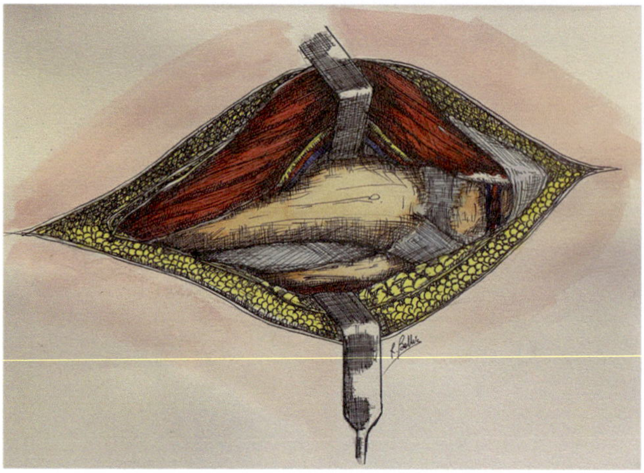

Fig. 17.4 Last exposition of distal tibia. © Rosa Ballis 2022. All Rights Reserved

17.3 Structures at Risk

- Just beneath the skin lies the superficial peroneal nerve (Fig. 17.2).
- Beware of anterior tibial artery and nerve.
- Deep peroneal nerve.

18 Posterolateral Distal Approach to the Leg

18.1 Introduction

Posterolateral approach of distal tibia is less commonly used as it is surgically more challenging. It offers good visualization of the posterior part of the tibia and fibula. In this chapter, we describe with text and images the posterolateral distal approach to the leg, tips and tricks and pitfalls.

- Indications: Fractures of distal part of posterior tibia.
- Position of the patient: Usually the patient is placed in prone or lateral position.
- Landmarks: Midline between distal fibula, lateral border of Achilles tendon and joint line.

18.2 Step-by-Step Procedure

– Incision: Skin incision is made between the lateral border of Achilles tendon and fibula and direction run from the tip of fibula distally and can be carried proximally as much as required (Fig. 18.1).

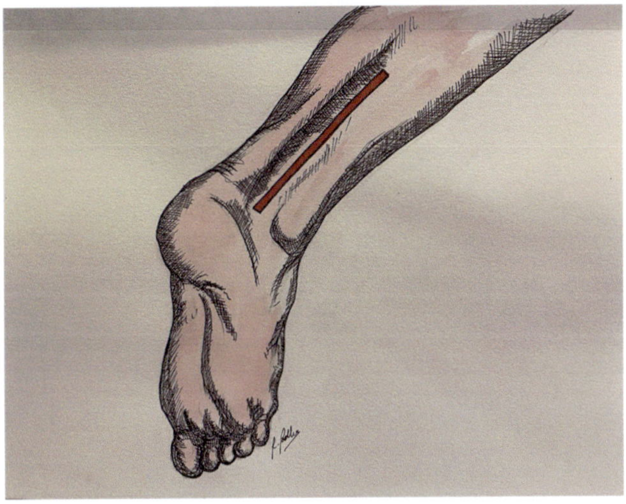

Fig. 18.1 Landmark incision. © Rosa Ballis 2022. All Rights Reserved

R. Ballis et al., *Atlas of Orthopaedic Surgical Approaches to the Lower Limbs*, https://doi.org/10.1007/978-3-031-07723-4_18

- After skin incision and dissection of the subcutaneous layer, the superficial peroneal nerve and the saphenous vein are identified.
- Aponeurosis incision is taken along skin incision (Fig. 18.2).
- Peroneus longus and brevis muscles are retracted laterally with its tendons like a lateral flap.
- Flexor hallucis longus muscle is retracted posteriorly (Figs. 18.3 and 18.4).
- Soleus muscle is detached from the periosteum.

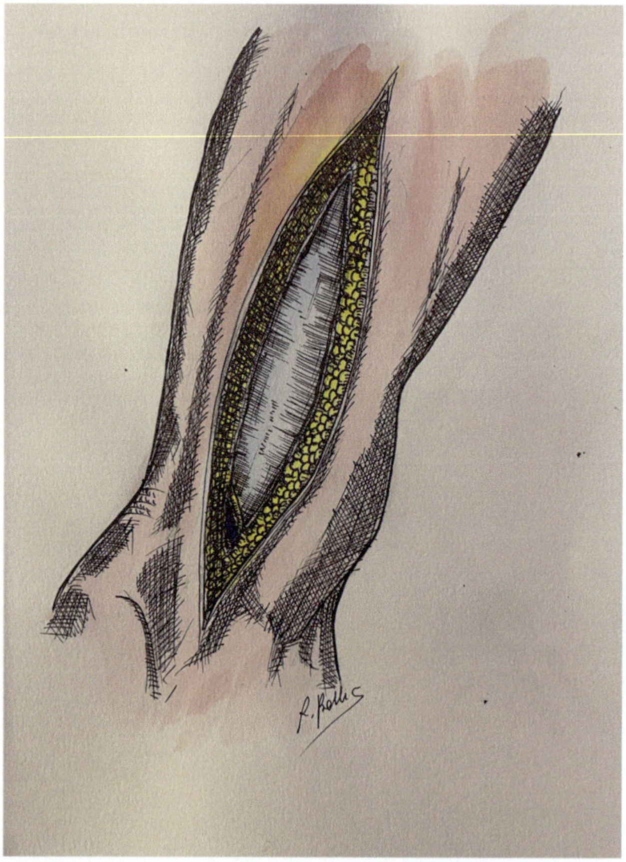

Fig. 18.2 Saphenous vein and superficial peroneal nerve.

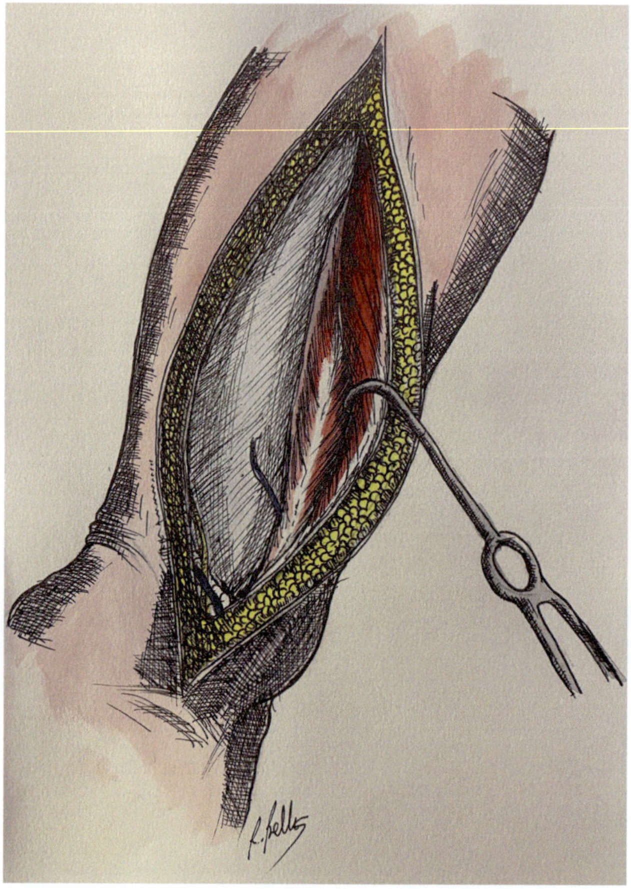

Fig. 18.3 Lateral retraction of peroneal muscles

- If a tibial exposition is needed, the flexor hallucis longus muscle is retracted laterally to protect the peroneal vessels and the flexor digitorum communis longus medially to protect tibial vessels and nerve (Figs. 18.5 and 18.6).

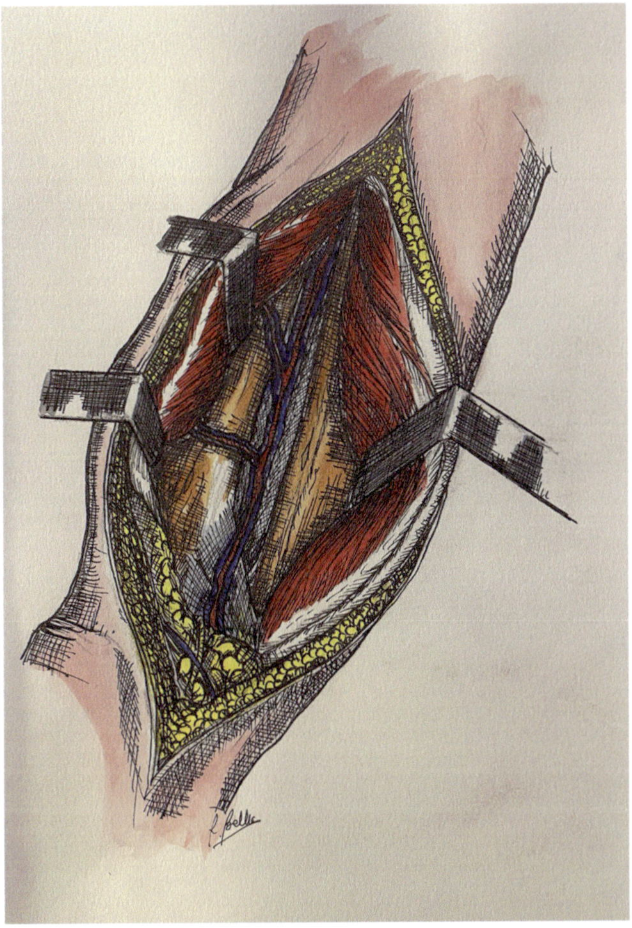

Fig. 18.4 Medial retraction of flexor hallucis longus and exposition of peroneal vessels. © Rosa Ballis 2022. All Rights Reserved

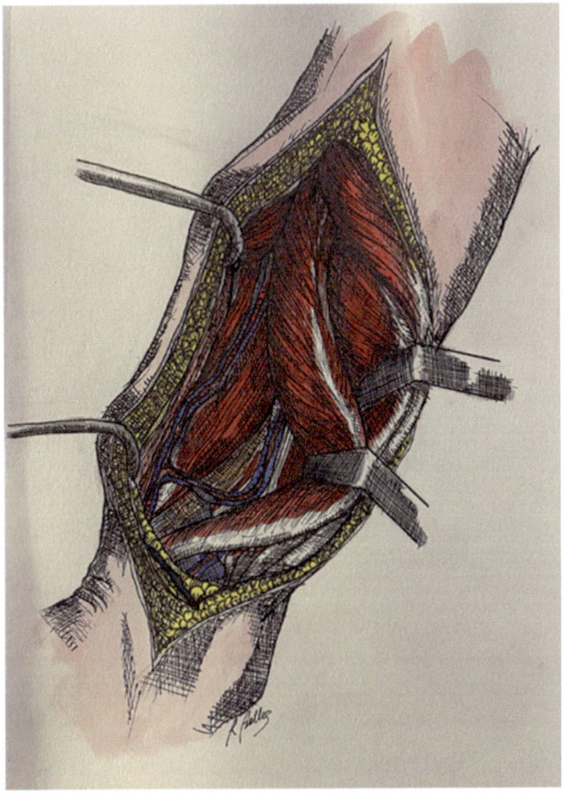

Fig. 18.5 Tibial exposition with retraction on flexor hallucis longus laterally. © Rosa Ballis 2022. All Rights Reserved

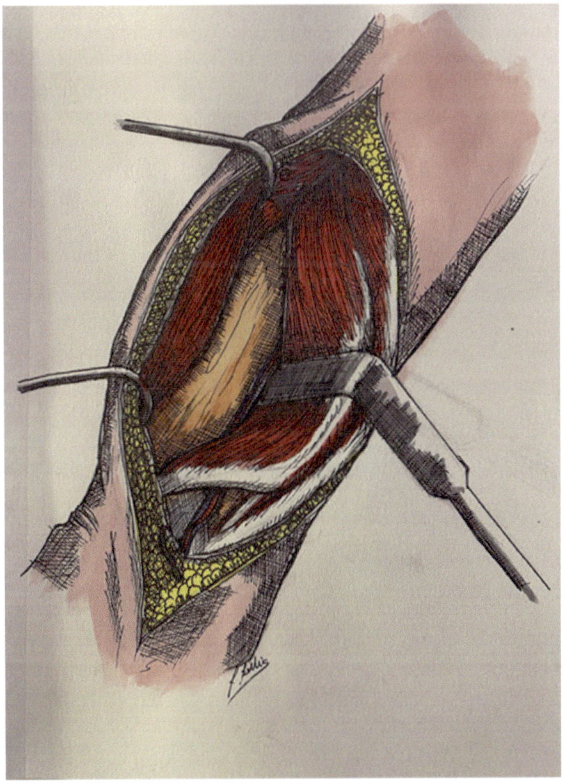

Fig. 18.6 Tibial exposure © Rosa Ballis 2022. All Rights Reserved

18.3 Structures at Risk

- Just beneath the superficial fascial layer proximally lies the superficial peroneal nerve.
- Posterior tibial vessels (protected by flexor hallucis longus).
- Sural nerve distally.
- Tibial nerve (protected by flexor hallucis longus).

Part IV

Ankle

19 Anatomy of the Ankle

19.1 Introduction

Ankle is a complex joint made up of two joints, the inferior talocrural joint and the subtalar joint. These joints are held together with three sets of ligaments. Muscles, tendons that control movement in ankle and foot and neurovascular structures that supply this region pass relatively superficial in the ankle area. A thorough knowledge of the anatomy of the ankle, is essential to perform safe and effective ankle surgery. Also this anatomical area presents problems in the peripheral vascularization for which incision and dissection of tissues must be performed with the utmost care. It is preferable to widen the incision rather than exert unnecessary tension in the skin, in order to avoid skin problems.

R. Ballis et al., *Atlas of Orthopaedic Surgical Approaches to the Lower Limbs*, https://doi.org/10.1007/978-3-031-07723-4_19

19.2 Lateral View

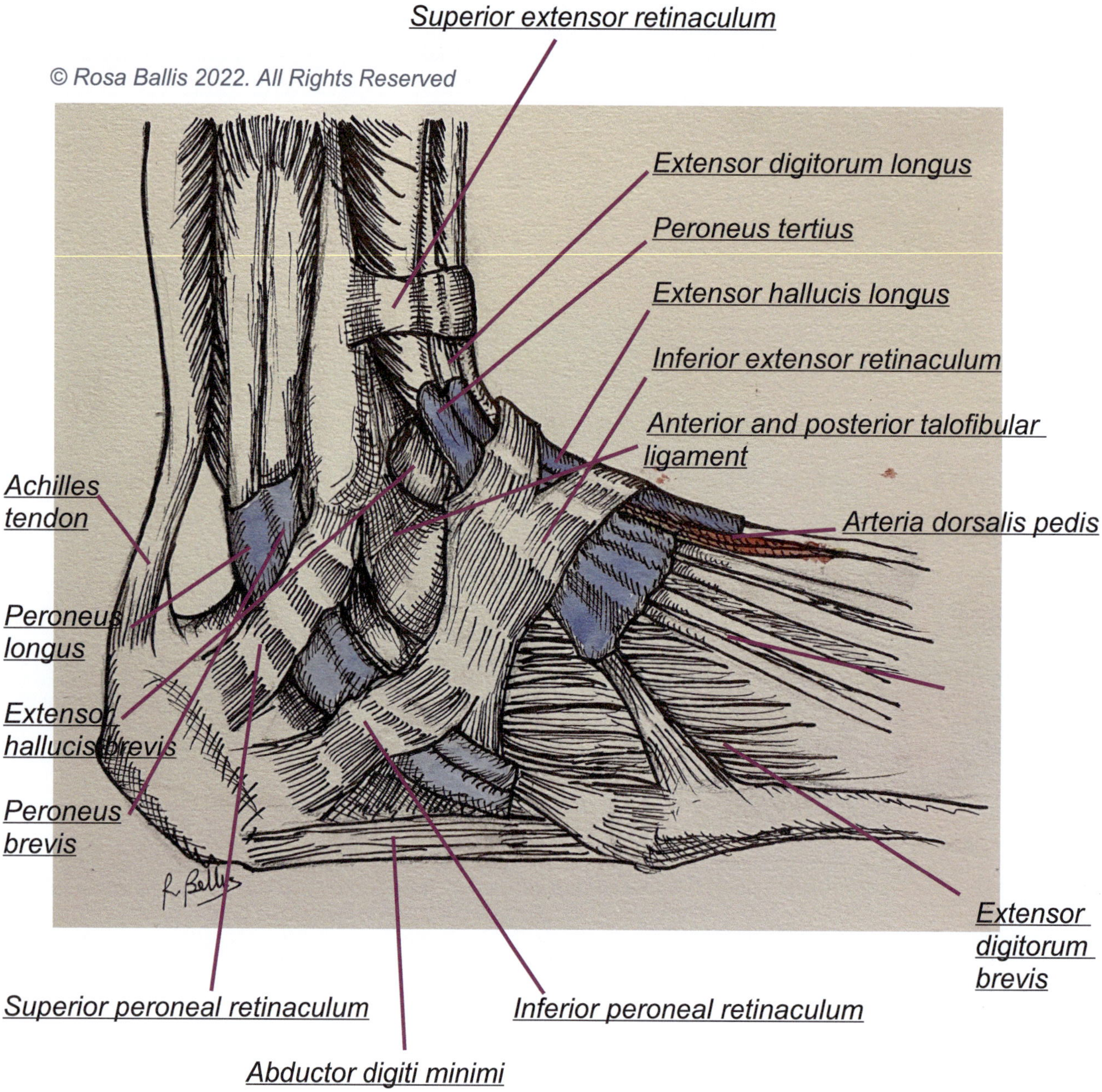

19.3 Medial View

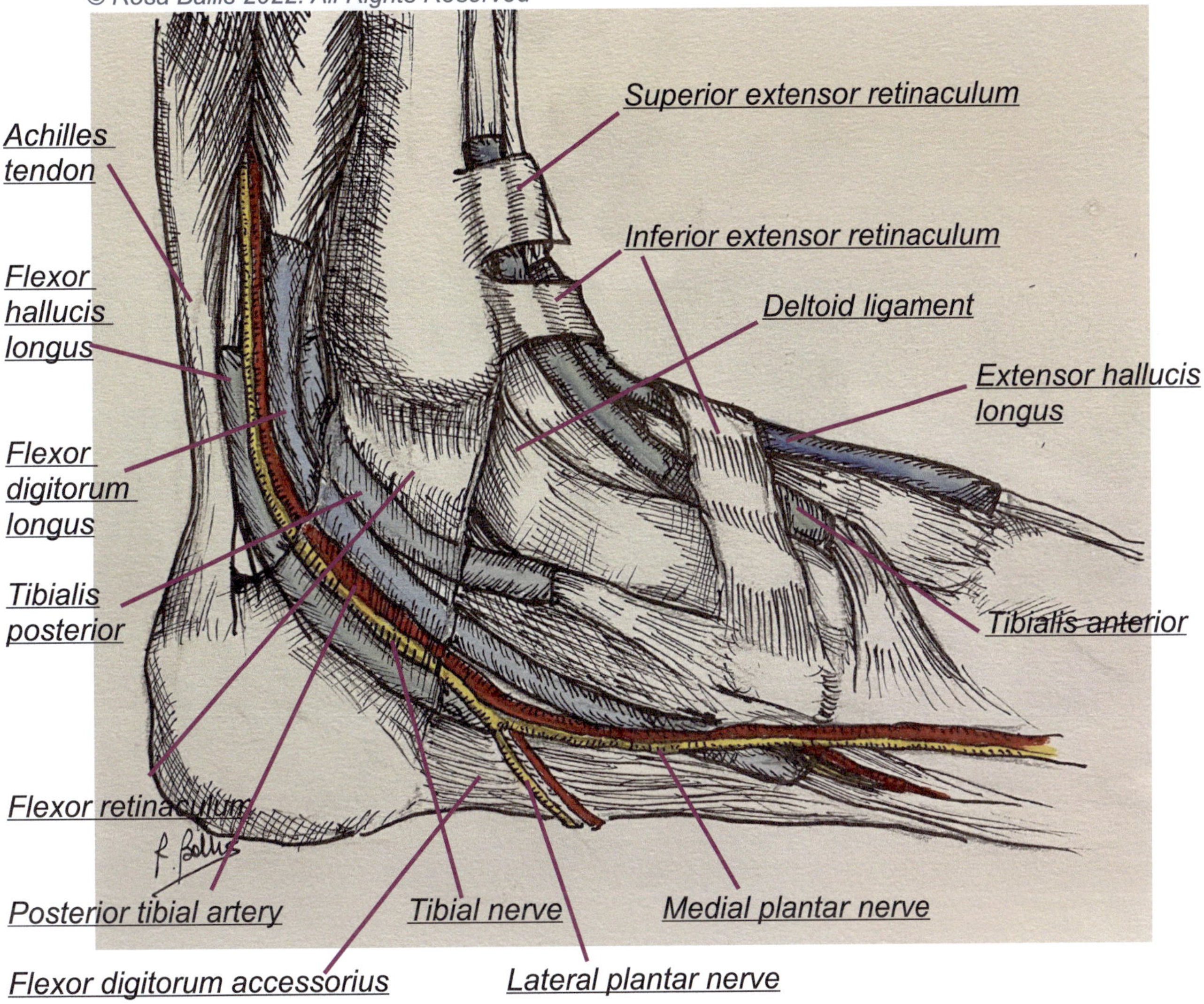

20 Lateral Approach to the Ankle

20.1 Introduction

The lateral approach to the ankle is used mostly for open reduction and internal fixation of lateral and third malleolous fractures. It offers visibility to the posterolateral aspect of the tibia.

- Indications: Fibular fractures, tumours, osteomyelitis.
- Position of the patient: Usually the patient is placed in supine position with a support under the homolateral hip to keep leg intrarotated.
- Landmarks: Tip and midline shaft of fibula.

20.2 Step-by-Step Procedure

– Incision: Longitudinal incision along the posterior edge of the fibula, to be continued as needed, 2 cm slightly anteriorly distal to tip of lateral malleoli (Fig. 20.1).

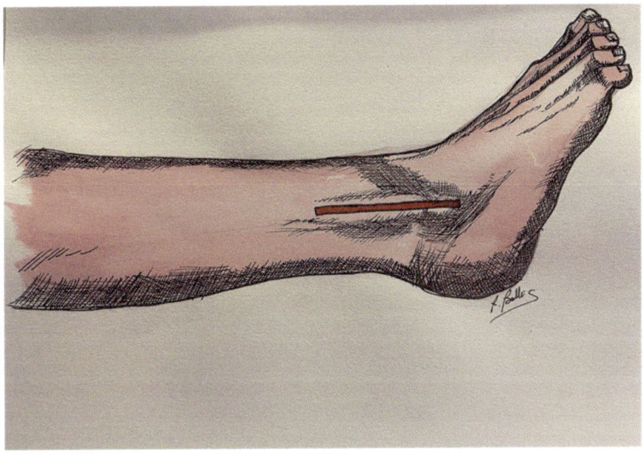

Fig. 20.1 Landmark incision. (© Rosa Ballis 2022. All Rights Reserved)

R. Ballis et al., *Atlas of Orthopaedic Surgical Approaches to the Lower Limbs*, https://doi.org/10.1007/978-3-031-07723-4_20

- Dissection is carried out between peroneus tertius anteriorly and peroneus longus and brevis posteriorly (Fig. 20.2).
- Periosteum is incised also longitudinally and the fibula is exposed (Fig. 20.3).

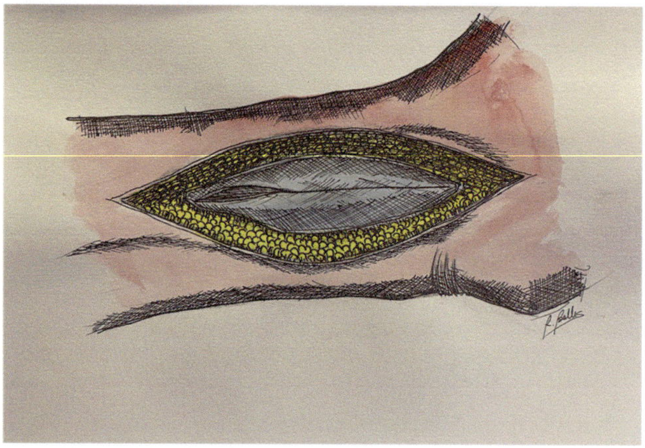

Fig. 20.2 Incision of the fascia under skin incision in the same line. (© Rosa Ballis 2022. All Rights Reserved)

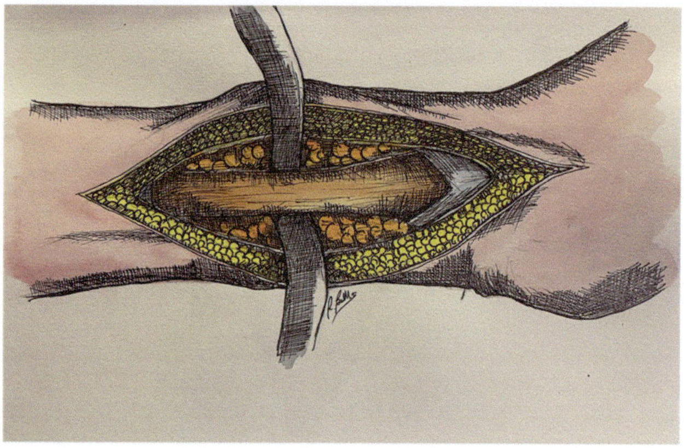

Fig. 20.3 Fibula exposure. (© Rosa Ballis 2022. All Rights Reserved)

20.3 Structures at Risk

- Take care to avoid short saphenous vein and sural nerve posteriorly and superficial peroneal nerve anteriorly to this incision.
- If incision is prolonged proximally, attention must be kept to peroneal muscles.

21 Medial Approach to the Ankle

21.1 Introduction

The medial approach of the ankle is used mostly for open reduction and internal fixation of medial malleolar fractures. It also offers access to the deltoid ligament for reparation.

- Indications: Fracture of the medial malleoli, deltoid ligament reconstruction.
- Position of the patient: Usually the patient is placed in supine position.
- Landmarks: Midline end of medial malleoli.

21.2 Step-by-Step Procedure

– Incision: Longitudinal, curved incision begins proximal to medial malleolus over subcutaneous tibia and continues across anterior third of medial malleolus (Fig. 21.1).

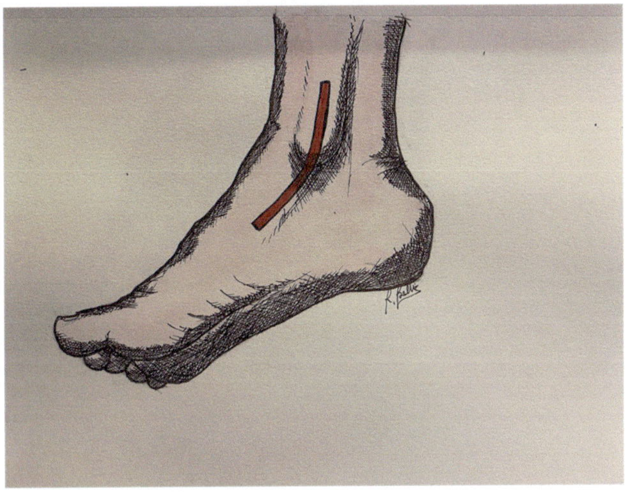

Fig. 21.1 Landmark incision. (© Rosa Ballis 2022. All Rights Reserved)

R. Ballis et al., *Atlas of Orthopaedic Surgical Approaches to the Lower Limbs*, https://doi.org/10.1007/978-3-031-07723-4_21

– Incision is carried out longitudinally along the periosteum, and medial malleoli is exposed (Fig. 21.2).

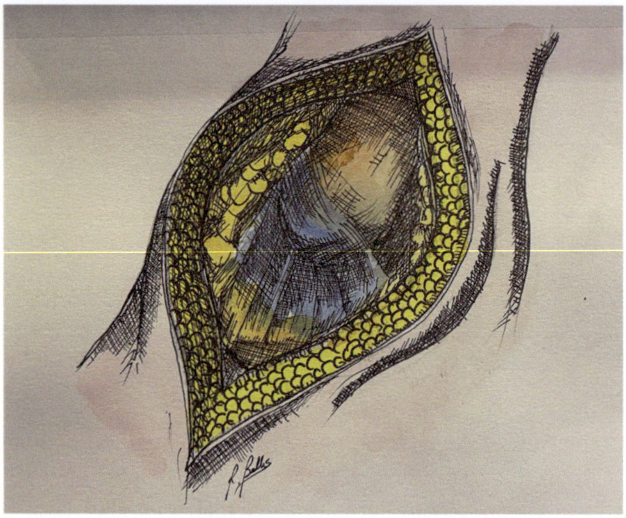

Fig. 21.2 Medial malleoli with deltoid ligament. (© Rosa Ballis 2022. All Rights Reserved)

21.3 Structures at Risk

- Long saphenous vein and nerve just anterior to medial malleolus must be protected.

Posterolateral Approach to the Ankle

22

22.1 Introduction

- Indications: Fracture of the distal part of tibia (Volkmann fragment) and fibula.
- Position of the patient: Usually the patient is placed in the prone or lateral position.
- Landmarks: Posterior edge of lateral malleoli, lateral border of Achilles tendon and joint line.

22.2 Step-by-Step Procedure

– Incision: Longitudinal incision is made between lateral malleoli and Achilles tendon and curved anteriorly for 2.5–4 cm in line with peroneal tendons (Fig. 22.1).

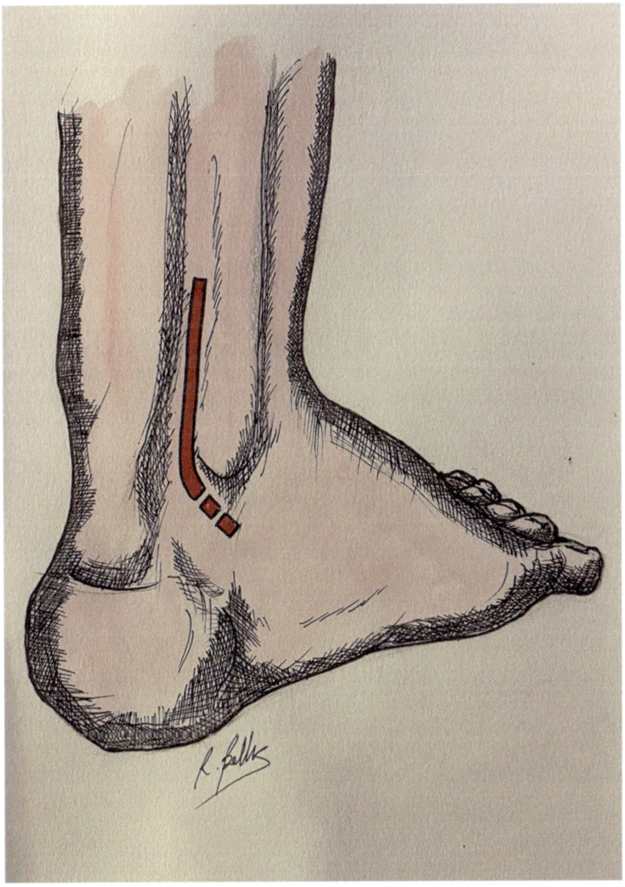

Fig. 22.1 Landmark incision. (© Rosa Ballis 2022. All Rights Reserved)

R. Ballis et al., *Atlas of Orthopaedic Surgical Approaches to the Lower Limbs*, https://doi.org/10.1007/978-3-031-07723-4_22

- When dissection arrives the fascia, beware of sural nerve in the medial side.
- Incision of the fascia is made between the flexor hallucis longus and the peroneus tendons (Fig. 22.2).
- For access in posterior malleoli:
  - Peroneal muscles are displaced laterally, peroneal tendon sheath is incised, and the tibial surface between flexor hallucis longus medially and the peroneal tendons laterally is exposed (Figs. 22.3 and 22.4).

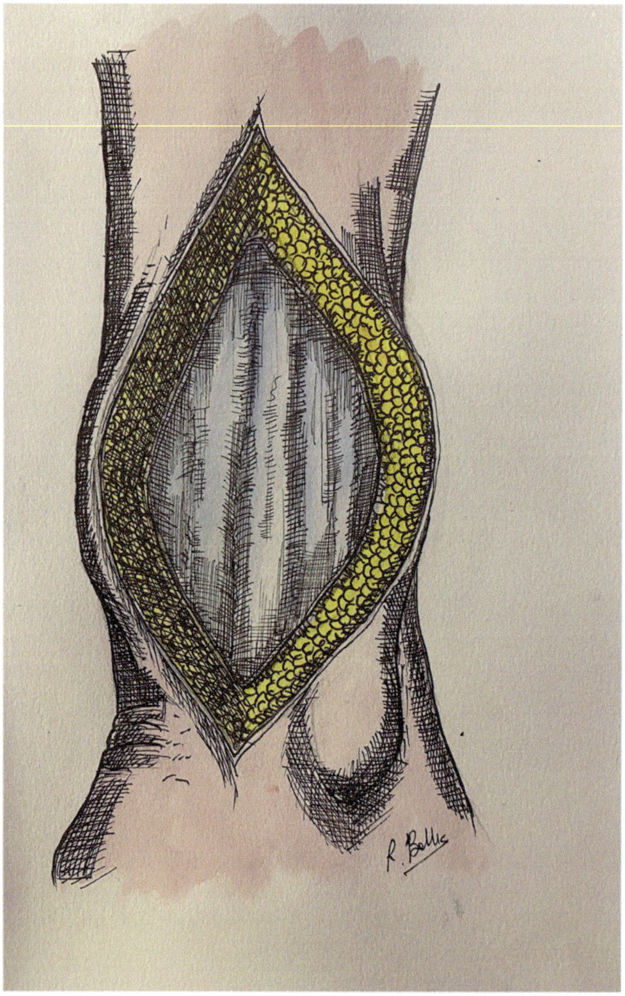

Fig. 22.2 The underneath fascia. (© Rosa Ballis 2022. All Rights Reserved)

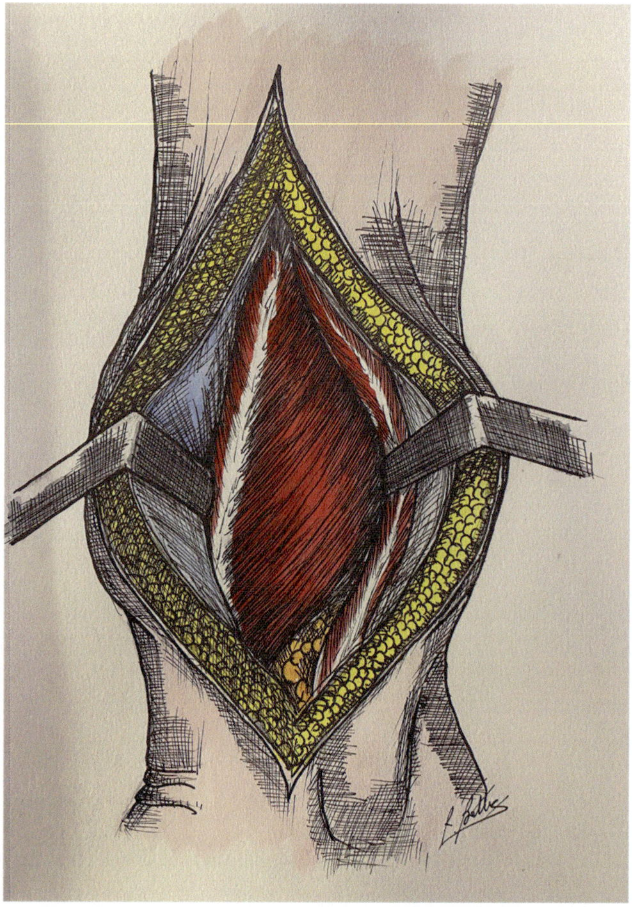

Fig. 22.3 Retraction of peroneal muscles. (© Rosa Ballis 2022. All Rights Reserved)

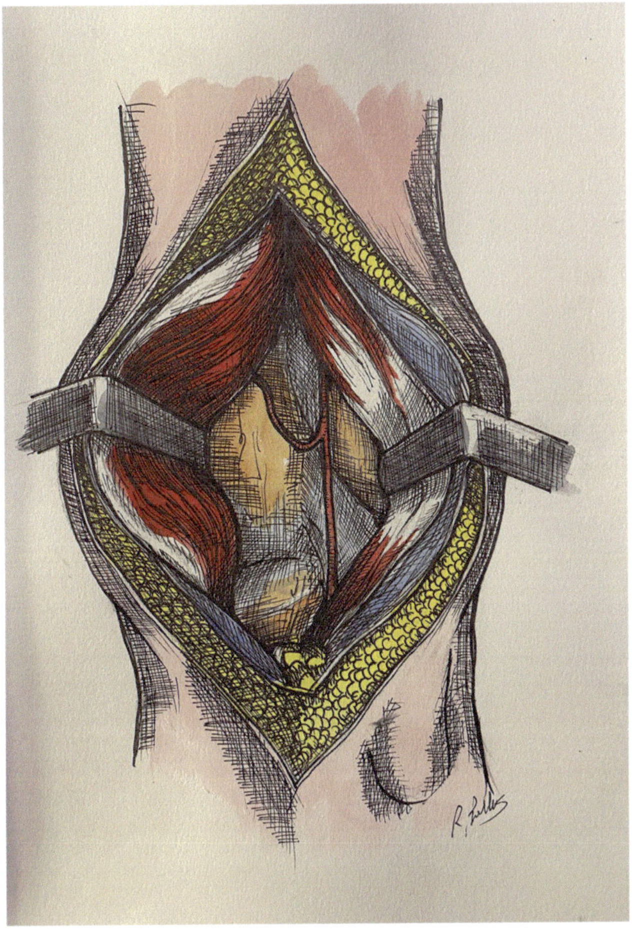

Fig. 22.4 Peroneal artery after complete retraction and tibia and posterior fibula exposure. (© Rosa Ballis 2022. All Rights Reserved)

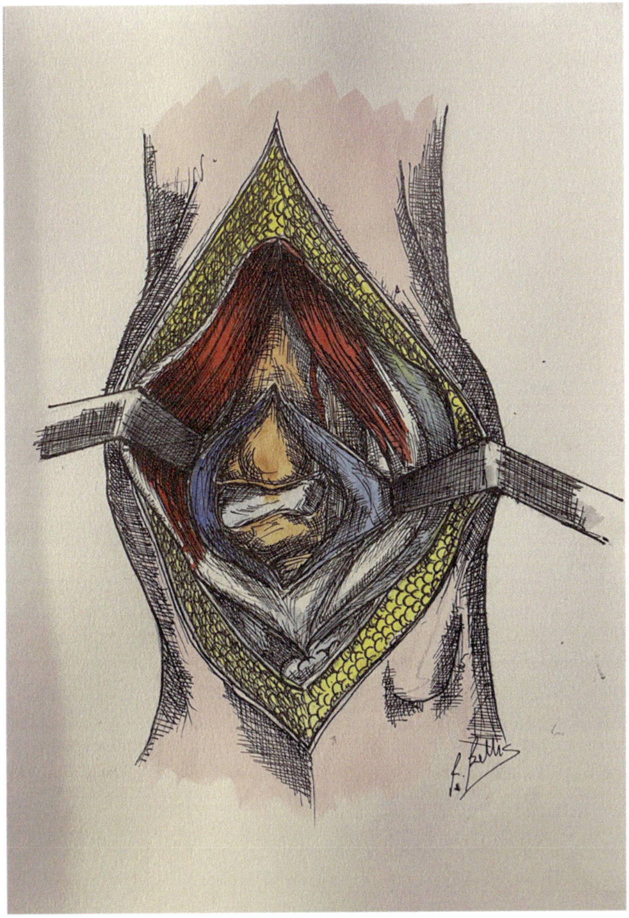

Fig. 22.5 Tibiotalar joint exposure. (© Rosa Ballis 2022. All Rights Reserved)

– For access in lateral malleoli:
  - Peroneal tendons are retracted medially.
  - Fibula is exposed including lateral malleolus subperiosteally.
– If access to tibiotalar joint is needed, dissection should proceed distally (Fig. 22.5).

22.3 Structure at Risk

- Sural nerve in the first part of dissection. It lies medially with the saphenous lateral vein.
- Peroneal artery laterally, attention must be paid to dissection.

23 Achilles Tendon Approach

23.1 Introduction

This approach is used for Achilles tendon repair, reconstruction or tendoplasty described with text and images.

- Indications: Achilles tendon repair, reconstruction or plasty.
- Position of the patient: Usually the patient is placed in prone position.
- Landmarks: Medial malleoli, medial border of Achilles tendon, calcanear insertion of Achilles tendon.

23.2 Step-by-Step Procedure

– Incision: Straight line medial to the Achilles tendon (Fig. 23.1).

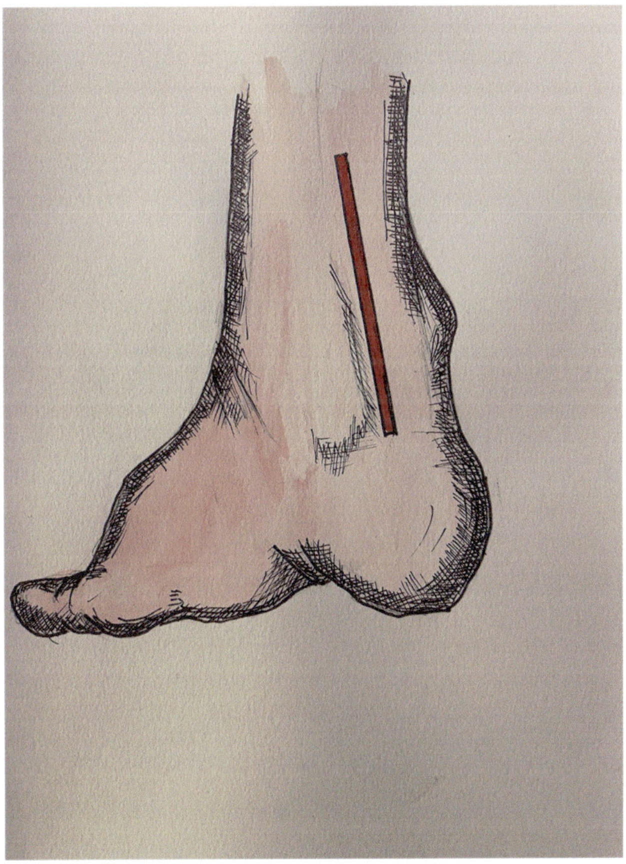

Fig. 23.1 Landmark incision. (© Rosa Ballis 2022. All Rights Reserved)

R. Ballis et al., *Atlas of Orthopaedic Surgical Approaches to the Lower Limbs*, https://doi.org/10.1007/978-3-031-07723-4_23

- Dissection must be performed carefully due to poor vascularization.
- Tendon lies immediately subcutaneous.
- Paratenon is incised, and tendon edges are exposed for repair (Figs. 23.2 and 23.3).

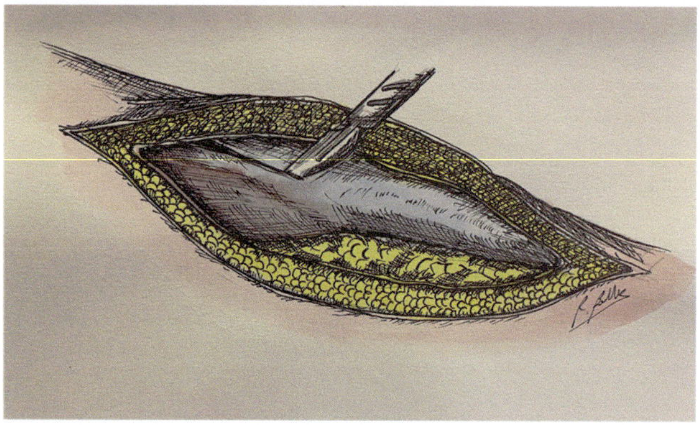

Fig. 23.2 Paratenon incision. (© Rosa Ballis 2022. All Rights Reserved)

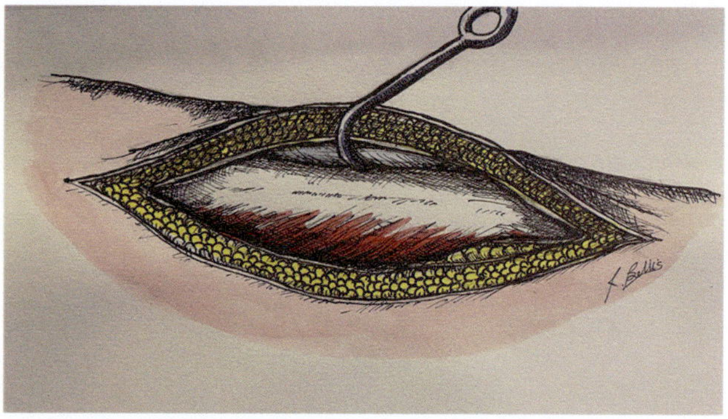

Fig. 23.3 Achilles tendon exposure. (© Rosa Ballis 2022. All Rights Reserved)

23.3 Structures at Risk

- The real danger consists of the regional poor vascularization. Incision and dissection should be performed carefully.
- In order to avoid damage to sural nerve, the incision in made medial to Achilles tendon.

References

1. Jordan CH, Mirzabeigi E. Atlas of orthopaedic surgical exposures. New York: Thieme; 2000.
2. Meermans G, Konan S, Das R, Volpin A, Haddad FS. The direct anterior approach in total hip arthroplasty: a systematic review of the literature. Bone Jt J. 2017;99(6):732–40. https://doi.org/10.1302/0301-620X.99B6.38053.
3. Lepri AC, Villano M, Matassi F, Carulli C, Innocenti M, Civinini R. "Anterolateral" approach to the hip: a systematic review of the correct definition of terms. Hip Int. 2020;30(2):13–9. https://doi.org/10.1177/1120700020966800.
4. Petis S, Howard JL, Lanting BL, Vasarhelyi EM. Surgical approach in primary total hip arthroplasty: anatomy, technique and clinical outcomes. Can J Surg. 2015;58(2):128–39. https://doi.org/10.1503/cjs.007214.
5. Parer MJ. Lateral versus posterior approach for insertion of hemiarthroplasties for hip fractures: a randomised trial of 216 patients. Injury. 2015;46(6):1023–7. https://doi.org/10.1016/j.injury.2015.02.020.
6. Cristea S, Predescu V, Dragosloveanu Ș, Cuculici Ș, Mărăndici N. Surgical approaches for total knee arthroplasty. London: IntechOpen; 2016.
7. Faucett SC, Gannon J, Chahla J, Ferrari MB, LaPrade RF. Posterior surgical approach to the knee. Arthrosc Tech. 2017;6(2):e391–5. https://doi.org/10.1016/j.eats.2016.10.013.
8. Berihu BA, Debeb YG. Anatomical variation in bifurcation and trifurcations of sciatic nerve and its clinical implications: in selected university in Ethiopia. BMC Res Notes. 2015;8:633.
9. Garner MR, Warner SJ, Lorich DG. Surgical approaches to posterolateral tibial plateau fractures. J Knee Surg. 2016;29:12–20.
10. Abbott LC, Carpenter WF. Surgical approaches to the knee joint. J Bone Joint Surg Am. 1974;27:227–310.
11. Mitsuzawa S, Takeuchi H, Ando M, Sakazaki T, Ikeguchi R, Matsuda S. Comparison of four posterior approaches of the ankle: a cadaveric study. OTA Int. 2020;3(3):e085. https://doi.org/10.1097/OI9.0000000000000085.
12. Lidder S, Masterson S, Grechenig S, et al. The risk of injury to the peroneal artery in the posterolateral approach to the distal tibia: a cadaver study. J Orthop Trauma. 2014;28:534–7.
13. Patzkowski JC, Kirk KL, Hsu JR, et al. Quantification of posterior ankle exposure through an Achilles tendon-splitting versus posterolateral approach. Foot Ankle Int. 2012;33:900–4.
14. Assal M, Ray A, Fasel JHD, et al. A modified posteromedial approach combined with extensile anterior for the treatment of complex tibial pilon fractures (AO/OTA 43-C). J Orthop Trauma. 2014;28:e138–45.
15. Femino JE, Vaseenon T. The direct lateral approach to the distal tibia and fibula: a single incision technique for distal tibial and pilon fractures. Iowa Orthop J. 2009;29:143–8.

R. Ballis et al., *Atlas of Orthopaedic Surgical Approaches to the Lower Limbs*, https://doi.org/10.1007/978-3-031-07723-4

MIX
Papier aus verantwortungsvollen Quellen
Paper from responsible sources
FSC® C105338

If you have any concerns about our products,
you can contact us on
ProductSafety@springernature.com

In case Publisher is established outside the EU,
the EU authorized representative is:
Springer Nature Customer Service Center GmbH
Europaplatz 3, 69115 Heidelberg, Germany

Printed by Libri Plureos GmbH
in Hamburg, Germany